T0215842

How to Read an EEG

How to Read an EEG

Neville M. Jadeja
University of Massachusetts Medical School

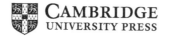

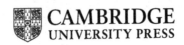

Shaftesbury Road, Cambridge CB2 8EA, United Kingdom

One Liberty Plaza, 20th Floor, New York, NY 10006, USA

477 Williamstown Road, Port Melbourne, VIC 3207, Australia

314–321, 3rd Floor, Plot 3, Splendor Forum, Jasola District Centre, New Delhi – 110025, India

103 Penang Road, #05–06/07, Visioncrest Commercial, Singapore 238467

Cambridge University Press is part of Cambridge University Press & Assessment,
a department of the University of Cambridge.

We share the University's mission to contribute to society through the pursuit of
education, learning and research at the highest international levels of excellence.

www.cambridge.org
Information on this title: www.cambridge.org/9781108825641

DOI: 10.1017/9781108918923

First published 2021

A catalogue record for this publication is available from the British Library

Library of Congress Cataloging-in-Publication data
Names: Jadeja, Neville M., 1986– author.
Title: How to read an EEG / Neville M. Jadeja.
Description: Cambridge, United Kingdom ; New York, NY : Cambridge
University Press, 2021. | Includes bibliographical references and index.
Identifiers: LCCN 2020052327 (print) | LCCN 2020052328 (ebook) | ISBN
9781108825641 (paperback) | ISBN 9781108918923 (ebook)
Subjects: MESH: Electroencephalography – methods | Brain
Diseases – diagnostic imaging | Electroencephalography – standards
Classification: LCC RC386.6.E43 (print) | LCC RC386.6.E43 (ebook) | NLM
WL 150 | DDC 616.8/047547–dc23
LC record available at https://lccn.loc.gov/2020052327
LC ebook record available at https://lccn.loc.gov/2020052328

ISBN   978-1-108-82564-1   Paperback

To Mia

Contents

Figure Contributions

Foreword

I have been learning and teaching the interpretation of electro-encephalograms for 20 wonderful years. It has been incredibly rewarding to learn how to use the tool of EEG, which is relatively inexpensive and safe, to improve the care of patients with seizures and other neurologic symptoms. I recommend that all neurologists try as much as possible to feel comfortable with the use of EEG and interpreting the reports of electroencephalographers. But, it can be challenging, and many clinicians wish they were better in this field. Dr. Neville Jadeja's book is a great place to start fulfilling this wish.

I had the pleasure of training Dr. Jadeja during his epilepsy fellowship at the Edward B. Bromfield Epilepsy Center at Brigham and Women's Hospital at Harvard Medical School. He has always shown a joy in both learning and teaching EEG. The reader should be aware that Dr. Jadeja's teaching always comes with a smile. When I read this book, I can hear his upbeat voice and even see that enthusiasm and sparkle in his eye that he brought to fellowship every day. In much of his teaching, I also hear the voice of my own mentor, Dr. Bromfield, who passed down his teaching to me and many of Dr. Jadeja's other teachers of EEG.

Dr. Jadeja is a true expert in reading EEGs. Beyond his fellowship with me, he completed a fellowship in neurophysiology and intraoperative monitoring at Massachusetts General Hospital and now works at the University of Massachusetts in the Epilepsy Division. Dr. Jadeja has used his expertise in EEG and teaching to write "a just right" EEG book for learning to read EEGs; it is not too lengthy and does not skip any important details. Honestly, learning to read an EEG can be a daunting proposition, but this book makes it easy and shows how practical a skill this can be. This book contains great images of EEGs as well as clear descriptions of typical findings in adults, children, and neurocritical care EEG monitoring. The section on writing a report is particularly helpful for the examples provided.

As an author of the Accreditation Council of Graduate Medical Education (ACGME) Neurology Milestones and Epilepsy Milestones,

I find it particularly noteworthy that Dr. Jadeja's book can fulfill all EEG-related neurology milestones. These milestones are explain an EEG in nontechnical terms, use appropriate terminology related to EEG, describe normal EEG features of wake and sleep states, recognize EEG patterns of status epilepticus, recognize common EEG artifacts, interpret common EEG abnormalities, create a report, and recognize normal EEG variants. Additionally, this book serves as excellent preparation and review for beginning advanced training in epilepsy and clinical neurophysiology.

For those looking to learn EEG for the first time and for those wishing to refresh your skills, this book is for you. Enjoy!

Tracey A. Milligan, MD, MS, FAAN
Epileptologist, Edward B. Bromfield Epilepsy Center
Vice Chair for Education, Department of Neurology,
Brigham and Women's Hospital

Director, Neurology Clinical Competency Committee, and Co-Director,
Neurology Fellowship Programs, Mass General Brigham
Assistant Professor of Neurology, Harvard Medical School

Preface

Electroencephalography (EEG) is a powerful test that can provide valuable insight into cerebral functioning. However, most clinicians, including neurologists who don't routinely read EEGs, find them complex and confusing. The lack of standardization among experienced electroencephalographers adds to this perception. Although many excellent atlases and reference texts exist, the need for a simple guide has been long felt. This book aims to fill that void with a stepwise approach. It enables readers, especially trainees, to confidently interpret EEGs and benefit their patients.

This approach borrows heavily from those of my teachers at the Edward B. Bromfield, MD comprehensive epilepsy program at the Brigham and Women's Hospital and the intra operative neurophysiology unit at Massachusetts General Hospital. I also gratefully acknowledge my clinical colleagues and technicians at the University of Massachusetts. I wish to thank Lenora Ocava, Peter Mabie, Mark Milstein and Matthew Robbins for inspiring me to study neurology and my colleagues Azad Irani, Jerestyn Khopoliwalla, Angeliki Vgontzas, Rachel Passannante, Kelsey Goostrey, Matthew Schrettner, Lu Lin, Claire Joubert, Kyle Rossi, Behnaz Esmaeli, Felicia Chu, Mugdha Mohanty, Minh Lang, Celia Gomes McGillivray, Ika Noviawaty, Jess Slammin and Don Chin for their encouragement. This book would have been impossible without the tolerance of my wife, Shilpa, and the support of our family and friends. Last but not least, I thank Anna Whiting, Camille-Lee Own, and Deborah van Wyk at Cambridge University Press for making this possible.

I hope you enjoy it.

How to Read This Book

This book has three parts that should be read sequentially.

Part I (Basics) equips the reader with the foundational knowledge necessary to begin reading EEGs. It consists of chapters dedicated to understanding the technical aspects of interpretation and the normal EEG.

Part II (Interpretation) is dedicated to EEG reading through a stepwise approach. This constitutes the heart of the book, with chapters about pattern recognition.

In Part III (Specific Conditions), there are EEG examples in specific clinical situations. This part reinforces the skills gained in Part II. It may also serve as a mini atlas during clinical practice. Mastery of this part enables the reader to clinically correlate the EEG to the indication for which it was requested.

Finally, there is an appendix dedicated to report writing.

Introduction

Electroencephalograms (EEGs) are ubiquitous in clinical neurology. They are used to evaluate transient neurological symptoms such as impaired awareness, altered sensations, or abnormal movements. They form a part of the evaluation of common neurological illness such as epilepsy, stroke, tumors, dementia, encephalopathy, and encephalitis. Their role in critical care medicine is increasingly being recognized. Neuroscience trainees can be sure to encounter them in the office, emergency room, at the bedside, and during various certification examinations. However, the level of comfort among trainees to confidently interpret EEGs is variable. At first, most trainees will be intimidated by their appearance and instinctively limit themselves to reading their reports. Misinterpretations of electrographic waveforms are also common resulting in needless suffering from misdiagnoses and medication misuse [1]. The best way to avoid these situations is to interpret the EEG yourself and understand its implications. Simply put, this book empowers you to do just that!

The aim of this chapter is to introduce the reader to the EEG through the following sections:

1. Basics
2. Indications
3. Limitations
4. Electrodes
5. Placing Electrodes (10–20 System)
6. Instrument
7. Display
8. Parameters
9. Calibration
10. Safety

Basics

History

In 1875, a British physiologist, Richard Caton first recorded "feeble currents of varying direction" through electrodes placed on the cortical surfaces. His work laid the ground work for electroencephalography. Later in 1929, Hans Berger, a German psychiatrist, recorded the first alpha rhythm (Berger waves) inventing the modern electroencephalogram. He was also the first to use it to study neurological disease [2]. In 1935, Gibbs, Davis, and Lennox first demonstrated the 3 Hz spike and wave of idiopathic generalized epilepsy (IGE), the subsequent year Gibbs and Jasper first reported interictal discharges in focal epilepsy [3,4]. The first EEG laboratory opened at Boston's Massachusetts General Hospital in 1936 [5]. Since then, the test has gained widespread use.

Biology

The main generators of electrographic activity are summations of excitatory and inhibitory postsynaptic potentials of pyramidal cells in the superficial layers of the cortex. Synaptic activity, unlike action potentials occurs constantly and is not an all or none response. Therefore, normal cerebral activity is continuous. Neurons are radially oriented in the cortex and generate radially oriented dipoles (opposing or polar charges). The superficial (outer) ends of these dipoles leads to tiny voltage fields on the scalp (potentials). The EEG records and displays the spatial distribution of these potentials and their variations with time [6]. Additional inputs from subcortical structures such as the thalamus and reticular activating system (RAS) synchronize neuronal activity and generate electrographic rhythms [7]. It is believed that at least 6–10 square centimeters of cortex (sizable area) is required to produce a waveform over the scalp. Therefore, smaller potentials or foci may be missed on scalp recordings [8].

Physics

Cortical neuronal activity generates scalp potentials. These potentials may be imagined to resemble mountain peaks. They are maximum at their focus and loose strength as distance from the source increases. Voltage is the difference in strength between two potentials (measured in microvolts or uV) and current is the flow of charge (electrons) between them (measured in milliamperes or mA). Like a river, current will flow from a region of higher potential (taller peak) to a region of lower potential (smaller peak). Resistance (measured in ohms) is the impediment encountered by the current during its flow. The relationship between voltage (V), current (I), and resistance (R) is governed by the equation $V = IR$ (Ohm's law) and forms the basic physical principle of recording EEGs.

The EEG machine measures and amplifies the strength and direction of the current between two electrodes (over two different potentials) and displays this as a waveform. The reader can interpret these waveforms to determine their location and significance when the recordings from pairs of electrodes (channels) are viewed on a display in standardized formations (montages) [9].

Indications

The EEG is inexpensive, readily available, painless, and noninvasive. Hence it is used in a wide variety of clinical settings. Furthermore, it has incredible temporal resolution. This means it changes almost instantly (milliseconds) with changes in cerebral activity. This is far superior than the very best scans which may take (at least) several minutes to show physiological changes.

For the reader's benefit, a few common indications are listed below.

Clinic

- Evaluate transient neurological spells or symptoms for potential seizures.
- Identify the risk of recurrence (epilepsy) after a first-time seizure.
- Define the type of epilepsy or syndrome.
- Investigate cognitive decline.

Wards (or Epilepsy Monitoring Unit)

- Capture and characterize neurological events.
- Potentially rule in or rule out epilepsy.
- Quantify and localize seizures.
- Guide epilepsy treatments including medication adjustments and surgery.
- Characterize sleep–wake states (sleep studies).

Emergency Room and Intensive Care Unit

- Diagnose and manage status epilepticus.
- Diagnose and differentiate encephalopathic states.
- Guide the titration of anesthesia and sedation.

Operating Room

- Intraoperative guidance in several neurosurgical and vascular procedures (such as carotid endarterectomy) [10].

Limitations

Despite all its advantages, the EEG has important technical and practical limitations.

Technical

Despite the best techniques (and intentions), recording cerebral activity from the scalp has limited spatial resolution. Each electrode samples a vast area of cortex, therefore it is not possible to precisely pinpoint the origin of cerebral waveforms but only estimate the general region. Furthermore, the dampening effect of thick skull bones makes scalp potentials very small (microvolts). They need to be amplified many hundreds of times over for display. Large amplifications may also result in heavy contamination from ambient electrical noise (60 Hz) and other types of artifact. Another issue is that the EEG in principle assumes the cortical surface as a smooth sphere but, the cortex is deeply in folded. Only about a third of the cortex (superficial gyri) is accessible for scalp recordings. Cortical potentials that are deep (sulcal), inferior (basal), or hidden (insular or mesial) have poor scalp signals [11].

Practical

The reader must understand that the EEG is a snap shot in time. Like a photograph of the ocean, it reflects the surf only at that point in time. It cannot predict future storms or calm seas. When seen, epileptiform abnormalities (discharges) may be associated with epilepsy, but they are not diagnostic of it. However, epileptiform abnormalities are more specific (about 95%) than sensitive (about 30%) for epilepsy. A small percentage of healthy adults (less than 1%) and a slightly higher percentage of healthy children (less than 4%) will have epileptiform abnormalities [12]. Less than a third of those with focal brain lesions will also have epileptiform abnormalities in the absence of clinical seizures [13]. Conversely, less than half of those with epilepsy have epileptiform abnormalities on a single scalp EEG. This yield is maximal within the first 24 hours or so after a seizure and decreases thereafter. The yield also improves with repeat studies, but it is never absolute. Also, the number of discharges correlates weakly with severity of the epilepsy or seizure focus [14]. Then there is the experience and skill of the reader themselves for which there is no substitute. Most readers will have some neuroscience background, but this is variable. Sleep – whether natural or after sleep deprivation increases an EEGs yield and every effort should be made to include it. So do activation procedures such as photic stimulation and hyperventilation. Increasing the duration of the recording with ambulatory EEG or long-term monitoring will further improve the sensitivity and specificity of the EEG. Recording a patient's seizures on long-term video EEG is considered the gold standard for confirmation of epilepsy [15,16].

Electrodes

Scalp electrodes are small cup shaped disks made of silver, gold or plastic coated with silver chloride. They have a flat rim with a 1 cm diameter and small hole in the central dome for electroconductive gel. This design allows the electrodes to fix on

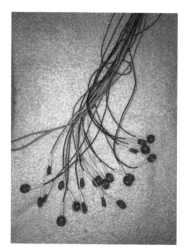

Figure 1.1 Scalp electrodes.

the scalp and effortlessly conduct electrical signals to the EEG machine. The electrode impedance (resistance to the flow of alternating current) must be less than 5 kohms. Higher impedances result in bad recordings. After carefully cleaning the scalp, electrodes are affixed with the help of small strips of gauze soaked in collodion or using electroconductive paste. If used, collodion is air-dried to form secure connections. Unprepared oily scalps result in higher impedance that distort the cerebral waveforms while sweat or gel bridges between electrodes result in lower impedances (short circuits) leading to artifact [17]. Figure 1.1 shows scalp electrodes.

Placing Electrodes (10–20 System)

Scalp electrodes must be placed on the scalp in a standardized fashion so that EEG recordings do not differ between laboratories. To achieve this, the "International 10–20 System of Electrode Placement" was developed by Dr. Herbert Jasper at the Montreal Neurological Institute in the 1950s and is accepted the world over with a few modifications [18].

According to this system, electrodes are placed on the scalp based on 10% or 20% increments of circumference measurements using easily identifiable skull landmarks. These are the nasion (top of the nose), inion (occiput), tragus, pinna, and mastoids. Each electrode position is described with a letter and a number. The letter indicates the underlying region the electrode records from (not exactly the lobe) such as prefrontal (Fp), frontal (F), temporal (T), parietal (P), occipital (O), and central (C). The number assigns its distance and position (right or left) of the midline (Z). Odd numbers overlie the left hemisphere and even numbers overlie the right hemisphere. A1 and A2 denote the left and right ear lobes (or mastoids). Figure 1.2 shows the typical 10–20 system arrangement.

1. The technician will first measure the longitudinal circumference of the head in the sagittal plane from nasion through the vertex (uppermost point of the head) to inion and this distance is considered 100%. Five points are marked along this line as follows – **Fpz** (10% from nasion), **Fz** (20% from Fp), **Cz** (20% from Fz), **Pz** (20% from Cz), and **Oz** (20% from Pz and 10% from inion) as shown in Figure 1.3.

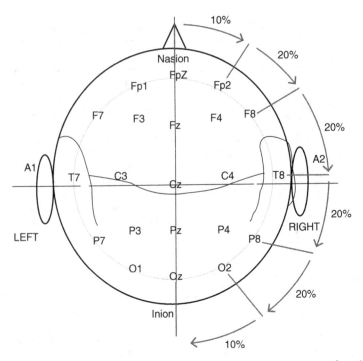

Figure 1.2 Electrode positions per the modified 10–20 system when viewed from the top of the head (not to scale).

2. Next, the transverse circumference is measured in the coronal plane from left to right preauricular points (root of the zygoma) through the vertex and this distance is considered a 100%. Seven points are marked along this line as follows – **A1** (Left preauricular point), **T7** (10% from left preauricular point), **C3** (20% from T7), **Cz** (20% from C3), **C4** (20% from Cz), **T8** (20% from C4), and **A2** (10% from T8 and at right preauricular point).

3. Then, a lateral circumference is measured from Fpz (anteriorly) to Oz (posteriorly), this passes through T7 on the left and T8 on the right. Points are marked (left/right) starting **Fp1/2** (10% from Fpz), **F7/8** (20% from Fp1/2), **T7/8** (20% from F7/8), **P7/8** (20% from T7/8), and **O1/2** (20% from P7/8 and 10% from Oz).

4. Finally, another parasagittal circumference is marked from Fp1 to O1 (through C3, left) and Fp2 to O2 (through C4, right) and considered 80% of the distance from Fpz to Oz. Three points are marked at 25% along this line as follows: **F3/4**, **C3/4**, and **P3/4**.

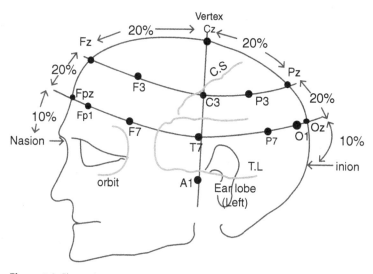

Figure 1.3 Electrode positions per the modified 10–20 system when viewed from the left side of the head (not to scale).

The system described here (modified combinatorial nomenclature) is an adaptation of the original 10–20 system as it renames four electrodes (T3 is T7, T4 is T8, T5 is P7, and T6 is P8) [19]. This conforms with the American Clinical Neurophysiology Society (ACNS) guidelines and is used in most EEGs in this book [20]. Some less commonly used placements include sphenoidal and nasopharyngeal electrodes. Sphenoidal electrodes are thin wires inserted through a needle placed between the zygoma and mandibular notch. They penetrate to a depth of 3 cm and may provide better resolution of anterior and mesial temporal structures [21]. Nasopharyngeal electrodes are placed through the nares into the posterior pharynx [22]. These placements are not routinely used as they are invasive and uncomfortable with debatable benefits.

Instrument

The EEG system amplifies and processes electrical signals recorded by pairs of scalp electrodes and displays these as waveforms on a digital screen. At its core are combinations of amplifiers called differential amplifiers. These additionally serve to reduce noise artifact between electrode pairs through common mode rejection by which the same artifact potential at both electrodes in each electrode pair will get cancelled out. However, for common mode rejection to work both electrodes in each electrode pair should be equally matched. If one of them is poorly fixed (high impedance) there is artifact in that channel. Scalp electrode impedances should be low for onward flow of current into the EEG system. Scalp electrode impedances should not exceed 5 kohms and impedance checks should be performed before each recording. Gain refers to the factor by which the signal is amplified and is measured in decibels (dB). Typically, a scalp signal needs to be amplified 1,000–100,000 times over (60–100 dB of voltage gain). Digital display systems will sample the amplified signal for storage and display. The sampling frequency refers to the number and density of data points sampled in time. Cerebral waveforms typically occur within 0.5 to 30 Hz frequency range so most digital displays will use a sampling frequency of 100 to 500 Hz to display representative waveforms [23]. A typical EEG set up consists of electrodes which must be applied to the patient's scalp. Each electrode has a wire connecting it to a headbox. The headbox is attached to a computer with a digital display screen using a thick cable. Figure 1.4 shows the parts of a typical EEG set up.

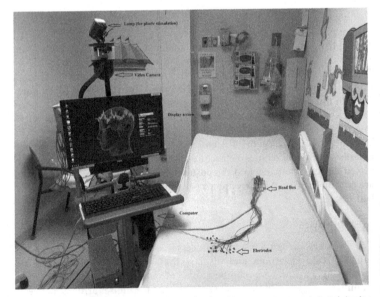

Figure 1.4 Typical EEG setup with electrodes, head box, computer, and digital display.

Display

There are a number of commercially available EEG systems. Readers must familiarize themselves with the individual nuances of the system used in their laboratory. For most displays, the top bar contains the recording parameters, montage, and other settings that can be easily changed per the reader's preference. A technologist's log may be pulled up to the right of the display. Most systems will show 10–15 s per page. Each major division (thicker lines) is 1 s within which there are five subdivisions (thinner lines) of 200 ms each. The EEG records in this book run at 15 s per page unless otherwise specified.

The appearance of the EEG will depend on its "montage." Most readers will default to the longitudinal bipolar montage (double banana) to begin their review. Most EEGs in this book are also shown in this montage. Figure 1.5 shows a typical display in the longitudinal bipolar montage.

The top four channels (each a pair of electrodes) are Fp1-F7, F7-T7, T7-P7, P7-O1. These record the patient's left temporal region in anterior to posterior direction (i.e., Fp1 is the anterior most electrode, and O1 is the posterior most in this chain).

The next four channels are Fp2-F8, F8-T8, T8-P8, P8-O2. These record the right temporal region in anterior to posterior direction. Placing these two sets in a staggered fashion allows the reader to easily compare both temporal activities.

Similarly, the following two sets compare the left paracentral Fp1-F3, F3-C3, C3-P3, P3-O1 and right paracentral Fp2-F4, F4-C4, C4-P4, P4-O2 regions. The bottom last two channels – Fz-Cz and Cz-Pz record over the midline. The final channel represents the electrocardiogram [EKG]. Other montages are described later in Chapter 3.

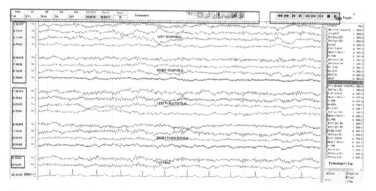

Figure 1.5 Typical appearance of an EEG display in longitudinal bipolar or double banana (DB) montage. Our laboratory uses a version of the Nihon Koden Workbench. Displays will vary depending on commercially available software in use.

Parameters

Sensitivity

The sensitivity (uV/mm) determines the magnification or size of the waveforms displayed. The reader can determine the strength of the potential (uV) as the product of its height (mm) and sensitivity (uV/mm). Readers will prefer a sensitivity of 7 uV/mm for most records. Low-voltage records may require a higher sensitivity. A maximum sensitivity of 2 uV/mm may be used to detect very low-voltage cerebral activity during brain death determinations. Lower sensitivities (such as 15 uV/mm) may be useful when reviewing higher amplitude waveforms such as spike waves to better appreciate their morphology.

Filters

The display allows filters to be applied to the signal. Clinically relevant cerebral activity lies between 0.5 to 50 Hz. Activity outside of this range (below or above) are potentially noise and may need to be filtered out to appreciate the underlying waveforms. At a filter cutoff frequency, at least 30% of that frequency is attenuated by filtration and the amount of attenuation exponentially increases above or below that frequency depending on the filter type. The time constant (t) is reciprocally related to the filter cutoff frequency. The reader should be familiar with three commonly used filters.

Low-Frequency Filter, LFF (High Pass): This filters out frequencies lower than the cutoff frequency allowing higher frequencies to pass. Standard LFF setting is 1 Hz (t 0.16 s). Low-frequency filters are useful in removing low-frequency contaminants such as pulsations, movements, and temperature related artifacts while preserving low-frequency detail such as slowing.

High-Frequency Filter, HFF (Low Pass): This filters out frequencies higher than the cutoff frequency allowing lower frequencies to pass. Standard HFF setting is 70 Hz. High-frequency filters are useful in removing high-frequency contaminants such as myogenic artifact while preserving high-frequency detail such as sharpness.

Notch filter is designed to specifically remove 60 Hz electrical noise.

Paper Speed

Most displays have their paper speed at 30 mm/s. Fast speeds (such as 60 mm/s) are useful to review high-frequency waveforms as they space out the closely packed activity while slower speeds (15 mm/s) may be useful for slow frequencies [24].

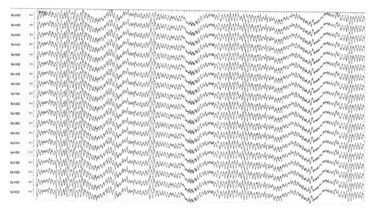

Figure 1.6 Nineteen-year-old man with epilepsy, bio calibration using Fp1-O2 channel.

Calibration Signal

The technologist should calibrate the EEG at the start and end of each recording. This allows the interpreter to confirm the sensitivity scale and integrity of the apparatus.

Initially, bio calibration may be performed where the patient themselves serve as a signal source and all channels use the same electrode pair (usually Fp1-O2 given the long interelectrode distance). In an awake patient, the posterior-dominant rhythm and blink artifact will be displayed in all channels confirming the ability of the EEG to record scalp signals. The technologist should check the responses for uniformity and make any adjustments necessary. Next, standard square wave calibration should be performed. At the usual sensitivity of 7 uV/mm, a calibration signal of 50 uV results in a deflection 7.1 mm in amplitude. The minimum recommended duration of recording is 20 min for adults and 60 min for neonates. Other requirements include having at least sixteen channels and three montages [24]. Figure 1.6 shows bio calibration, and Figure 1.7 shows square wave calibration.

Safety

As with other medical devices, the EEG machine is periodically inspected by the hospital's biomedical engineering department to ensure compliance with safety standards. The machine should also have a common ground that is isolated from the patient to avoid accidental electrocution and reduce artifact. Collodion is flammable and should be stored and handled safely. Prolonged application of EEG electrodes may result in skin erosion [25]. Periodic skin

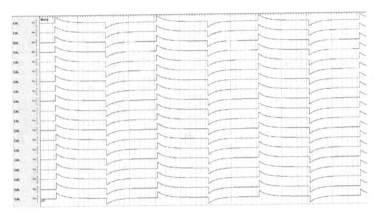

Figure 1.7 Same patient in Figure 1.6, square wave calibration using a 50 uV calibration signal.

safety checks are recommended for those on long-term EEG monitoring. Hospital infection control guidelines must be routinely followed. Disposable electrodes should be used when prion disease (such as Creutzfeldt–Jakob disease) is suspected and properly discarded thereafter [26].

Chapter Summary

1. EEGs are a simple and commonly used neurological test that most trainees find hard to interpret.
2. Summations of excitatory and inhibitory postsynaptic potentials of pyramidal neurons in the superficial layers of the cortex generate electrographic activity. These occur constantly, hence normal electrographic activity is continuous.
3. Subcortical structures such as the thalamus and reticular activating system (RAS) modulate cortical neuronal activity, resulting in electrographic rhythms.
4. A sizable area of cortex is required to generate enough signal on scalp recordings. Small potentials may be missed.
5. Voltage is current times resistance (Ohm's law).
6. EEGs are used in a variety of clinical care settings, including the clinics, wards, emergency rooms, critical care units, and operating rooms.
7. Like every other test, the EEG has technical and practical limitations.
8. EEG electrodes should have low impendences (less than 5 kohms).

9. Electrodes are placed on the scalp using a standardized system (international 10–20 system).
10. EEGs should be calibrated before and after each recording. Impedance should be checked.
11. Each major division is 1 s, within which there are five subdivisions of 200 ms each.
12. For adult records, most readers will use a sensitivity of 7 uV/mm, a low-frequency filter of 1 Hz, a high-frequency filter of 70 Hz, a notch filter (60 Hz), and paper speed of 30 mm/s.

References

1. Benbadis SR, Tatum WO. Overintepretation of EEGs and misdiagnosis of epilepsy. *Journal of Clinical Neurophysiology.* 2003 Feb 1;**20**(1):42–4.

2. La Vaque TJ. The history of EEG Hans Berger: psychophysiologist. A historical vignette. *Journal of Neurotherapy.* 1999 Apr 1;**3**(2):1–9.

3. Pearl PL, Holmes GL. Childhood absence epilepsies. In *Pediatric epilepsy: Diagnosis and therapy* (pp. 323–34). Demos Medical Publishing, New York; 2008.

4. Jasper H, Kershman J. Electroencephalographic classification of the epilepsies. *Archives of Neurology and Psychiatry.* 1941 Jun 1;**45**(6):903–43.

5. Barlow JS. The early history of EEG data-processing at the Massachusetts Institute of Technology and the Massachusetts General Hospital. *International Journal of Psychophysiology.* 1997 Jun 1;**26**(1–3):443–54.

6. Wong PK. Potential fields, EEG maps, and cortical spike generators. *Electroencephalography and Clinical Neurophysiology.* 1998 Feb 1;**106**(2):138–41.

7. Hughes SW, Crunelli V. Thalamic mechanisms of EEG alpha rhythms and their pathological implications. *The Neuroscientist.* 2005 Aug;**11**(4):357–72.

8. Cooper R, Winter AL, Crow HJ, Walter WG. Comparison of subcortical, cortical and scalp activity using chronically indwelling electrodes in man. *Electroencephalography and Clinical Neurophysiology.* 1965 Feb 1;**18**(3):217–28.

9. Jackson AF, Bolger DJ. The neurophysiological bases of EEG and EEG measurement: A review for the rest of us. *Psychophysiology.* 2014 Nov;**51**(11):1061–71.

10. Herman ST, Abend NS, Bleck TP, et al. Consensus statement on continuous EEG in critically ill adults and children, part I: indications. *Journal of Clinical Neurophysiology.* 2015 Apr;**32**(2):87.

11. Worrell GA, Lagerlund TD, Buchhalter JR. Role and limitations of routine and ambulatory scalp electroencephalography in diagnosing and managing seizures. *Mayo Clinic Proceedings.* 2002 Sep 1;**77**(9):991–8.

12. Cavazzuti GB, Cappella L, Nalin A. Longitudinal study of epileptiform EEG patterns in normal children. *Epilepsia*. 1980 Feb;21(1):43–55.

13. Pohlmann-Eden B, Hoch DB, Cochius JI, Chiappa KH. Periodic lateralized epileptiform discharges – a critical review. *Journal of Clinical Neurophysiology*. 1996 Nov 1;13(6):519–30.

14. Salinsky M, Kanter R, Dasheiff RM. Effectiveness of multiple EEGs in supporting the diagnosis of epilepsy: an operational curve. *Epilepsia*. 1987 Aug;28(4):331–4.

15. Veldhuizen R, Binnie CD, Beintema DJ. The effect of sleep deprivation on the EEG in epilepsy. *Electroencephalography and Clinical Neurophysiology*. 1983 May 1;55(5):505–12.

16. Fowle AJ, Binnie CD. Uses and abuses of the EEG in epilepsy. *Epilepsia*. 2000 Mar;41:S10–18.

17. Ferree TC, Luu P, Russell GS, Tucker DM. Scalp electrode impedance, infection risk, and EEG data quality. *Clinical Neurophysiology*. 2001 Mar 1;112(3):536–44.

18. Homan RW, Herman J, Purdy P. Cerebral location of international 10–20 system electrode placement. *Electroencephalography and Clinical Neurophysiology*. 1987 Apr 1;66(4):376–82.

19. Seeck M, Koessler L, Bast T, et al. The standardized EEG electrode array of the IFCN. *Clinical Neurophysiology*. 2017 Oct 1;128(10):2070–7.

20. Acharya JN, Hani AJ, Cheek J, Thirumala P, Tsuchida TN. American Clinical Neurophysiology Society guideline 2: guidelines for standard electrode position nomenclature. *The Neurodiagnostic Journal*. 2016 Oct 1;56(4):245–52.

21. Sperling MR, Engel Jr J. Sphenoidal electrodes. *Journal of Clinical Neurophysiology*. 1986 Jan 1;3(1):67–73.

22. DeJesus PV, Masland WS. The role of nasopharyngeal electrodes in clinical electroencephalography. *Neurology*. 1970 Sep 1;20(9):869.

23. Teplan M. Fundamentals of EEG measurement. *Measurement Science Review*. 2002 Jan;2(2):1.

24. Sinha SR, Sullivan LR, Sabau D, et al. American clinical neurophysiology society guideline 1: minimum technical requirements for performing clinical electroencephalography. *The Neurodiagnostic Journal*. 2016 Oct 1;56(4):235–44.

25. Drees C, Makic MB, Case K, et al. Skin irritation during video-EEG monitoring. *The Neurodiagnostic Journal*. 2016 Jul 2;56(3):139–50.

26. Cyngiser TA. Creutzfeldt–Jakob disease: a disease overview. *American Journal of Electroneurodiagnostic Technology*. 2008 Sep 1;48(3):199–208.

Polarity

The EEG display consists of an arrangement of channels.

Each channel is made up of two individual recording electrodes that are glued to the patient's scalp and record the electrical activity of the underlying cortex. The EEG machine constantly calculates the difference in electrical potential between these two electrodes, amplifies and then displays it as a deflection (wave) on the screen.

For example, if E1 and E2 are two scalp electrodes that make up channel E1-E2, then the direction and amplitude of the wave displayed by channel E1-E2 depends on the relative difference in electrical potentials at E1 and E2 (E1-E2).

Conventionally,

1. if the potential at E1 is less than E2 (E1 is relatively negative) then their difference (E1-E2) will be negative – manifesting as an upward deflection;
2. if the potential at E2 is less than E1 (E2 relatively negative) then their difference (E1-E2) will be positive – manifesting as a downward deflection;
3. if both E1 and E2 are equipotential or inactive (E1 = E2) then their difference (E1-E2) will be neutral – manifesting as no deflection.

Therefore, the display pointer always deflects toward the relatively smaller (more negative/less positive) electrode. If this electrode is E1, the deflection is upward (negative) and if it is E2, the deflection is downward (positive). If both electrode potentials are equal or inactive, there is no deflection [1]. Figure 2.1 illustrates polarity.

Chapter Summary

1. The polarity (direction and amplitude of deflection) depends on the relative difference between the two electrode potentials.
2. The pointer always deflects to the electrode with the relatively smaller potential (more negative/less positive).

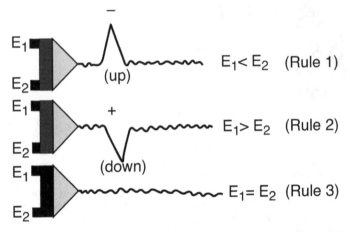

Figure 2.1 Upward (negative), downward (positive), and no deflection (neutral).

3. Upward deflection is surface negative, and downward deflection is surface positive.

Reference

1. Niedermeyer E. The EEG signal: polarity and field determination. In Electroencephalography: basic principles, clinical applications, and related fields (pp. 79–83). Oxford University Press, Oxford; 1987.

Chapter 3

Montages

The specific arrangement of channels (electrode pairs) on an EEG display is called a *montage* (French for "assembly"). This arrangement of channels allows the reader to analyze a waveform from a specific point of view. The reader may conceptualize montages to resemble the cuts of a head scan (such as axial, sagittal, or coronal) as each montage observes the same electrographic activity from a specific angle. Multiple designs exist but overall, montages can be grouped into one of two basic types:

1. bipolar
2. referential

Bipolar montages record the difference in potential between two adjacent electrodes. Both these electrodes intend to measure cortical electrical activity, that is, both are active electrodes. Bipolar montages are named based on the plane their electrode pairs are arranged. Longitudinal bipolar montage (also called a double banana based on its resemblance) and transverse bipolar montages are the two most commonly used bipolar montages [1]. As described earlier, most of the EEGs in this book use this montage. Other types of bipolar montages include the coronal and circumferential montages. Their advantages are explained later in Chapter 4. Figure 3.1 shows the display (A) and diagram (B) of electrode pairs in a longitudinal bipolar montage while Figure 3.2 shows the display (A) and diagram (B) of electrode pairs in a transverse montage.

Referential montages record the difference in potential between two distant electrodes. One of the two electrodes is active (records cerebral activity) while the other, relatively inactive electrode, is intended to serve as a "reference." The ipsilateral, contralateral ear or vertex are commonly used points of references as these are usually neutral. The computed average potential of all the active electrodes may also be used as a hypothetical reference point (average reference) [1]. Figure 3.3 shows the display (A) and diagram (B) of electrode pairs in an ipsilateral ear reference montage while Figure 3.4 shows the display of an average reference montage.

(A)

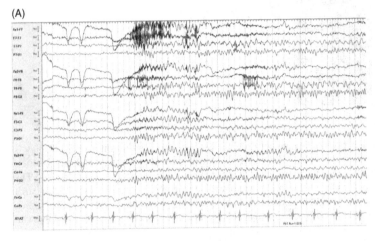

(B)

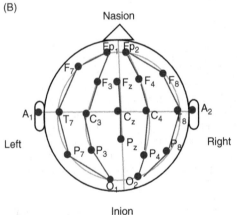

Figure 3.1 (A) Twenty-nine-year-old man with epilepsy, EEG display in longitudinal bipolar montage. This is also the default montage used to display EEGs in this book. (B) Diagram of electrode pairs used in the longitudinal bipolar montage.

Each montage has its distinct strength and weakness. Waveforms of interest should be viewed using both types of montages for accurate localization. Digital displays allow the reader to easily switch between different montages. At the minimum, every EEG must have a longitudinal and transverse bipolar as well as a referential montage [1].

(A)

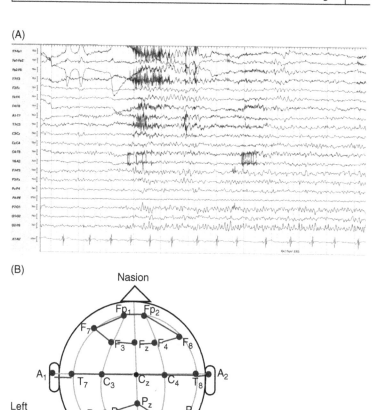

(B)

Figure 3.2 (A) Same patient as in Figure 3.1A, EEG display in transverse bipolar montage. (B) Diagram of electrode pairs used in the transverse bipolar montage.

Strengths and Weaknesses

Bipolar montages: As the electrodes in a bipolar montage are adjacent to each other, these montages offer the best "resolution" for focal potentials such as discharges. Another advantage is that they are usually less prone to artifactual

(A)

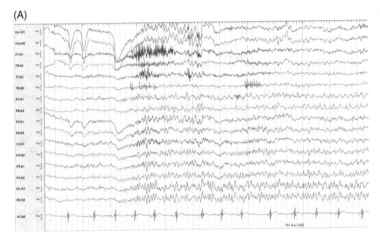

(B)

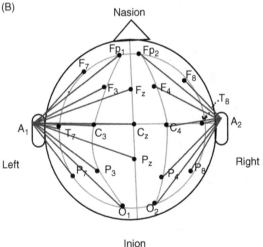

Figure 3.3 (A) Same patient as in Figure 3.1A, EEG display in an ipsilateral ear reference montage. (B) Diagram of electrode pairs used in the ipsilateral ear reference montage.

contamination. This is because artifactual potentials tend to involve adjacent electrodes to a similar degree and thus neutralize each other. On the flip side, their main disadvantage pertains to poor resolution for broad or generalized

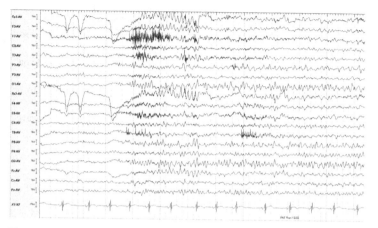

Figure 3.4 Same patient as in Figure 3.1A, EEG display in the average reference montage.

potentials. Since these are thinly spread out over a large area, there is only a small potential difference between adjacent electrodes. Therefore, broad or generalized potentials are much harder to appreciate on a bipolar montage.

Referential montage: As the electrodes are far apart, these montages offer the best "resolution" for broad or generalized potentials. Small potential differences are amplified with longer interelectrode distances. On the flip side, referential montages are prone to artifactual contamination as a contaminated reference leads to artifact in all the channels [2]. Understanding montages is the key to successful localization.

Chapter Summary

1. Montages are specific arrangements of channels; a channel is a pair of electrodes.
2. Waveforms result from cerebral potentials; each montage allows the reader to appreciate the same waveform through a distinct point of view.
3. Bipolar montages consist of channels with adjacent electrode pairs.
4. Referential montages consist of channels with nonadjacent electrode pairs. One electrode is located closer to the cerebral activity (active), while the other is intended as a distant reference (inactive).
5. Common bipolar montages include the longitudinal bipolar (double banana) and transverse bipolar.

6. Common referential montages include contralateral and ipsilateral ear reference, central reference (vertex), or average reference.
7. Bipolar montages are less prone to artifact and best appreciate focal potentials.
8. Referential montages are more prone to artifact and best appreciate broad or generalized potentials.
9. An active reference results when the reference which is intended to be neutral is very active.
10. The reader must use both types of montages to evaluate the same waveform. Digital displays make it easy to switch between montages.

References

1. Sinha SR, Sullivan LR, Sabau D, et al. American clinical neurophysiology society guideline 1: minimum technical requirements for performing clinical electroencephalography. *The Neurodiagnostic Journal.* 2016 Oct 1;56(4):235–44.

2. Britton JW, Frey LC, Hopp JL, et al. *Electroencephalography (EEG): an introductory text and atlas of normal and abnormal findings in adults, children, and infants.* American Epilepsy Society, Chicago; 2016.

Localization

Localization is the art of estimating the site of the maximum potential (origin of a waveform on the cortex). This depends on the montage in use and the rule of polarity, that is, the pointer deflects toward the relatively negative electrode.

Using different montages, the reader can roughly estimate the location of a waveform but unlike imaging, this technique is presumptive and imprecise. It assumes that the cortex is a smooth sphere with all its potentials arranged in the form of radial spokes. Each potential is a dipole with a superficial end that lends itself recordable from a surface electrode and a deep end that is not recordable. Of course, we know that the cortex is neither smooth nor spherical and therefore occult potentials often exist over sites such as the depths of a sulcus, inferior frontal lobes or insula that may not be detected by scalp EEG [1].

Localization Using a Bipolar Montage

Phase reversal is the key to localizing a waveform in a bipolar montage. This is the simultaneous but opposite deflection of the waveform in two channels that contain a common electrode. It implies that the potential is maximal at or near the location of the common electrode. If a longitudinal bipolar montage is in use, the next step would be to confirm the location of the phase reversal using another bipolar montage oriented perpendicular to the initial montage such as a transverse bipolar montage. Most phase reversals are negative (><), though positive phase reversals (<>) may also occur (especially in children). As mentioned previously, bipolar montages are best suited for detecting focal and not broad or generalized potentials [2]. Figure 4.1 explains the formation of a phase reversal in longitudinal bipolar montage over a hypothetical potential.

Localization Using a Referential Montage

The greatest amplitude of the deflection is key to localizing a waveform in a referential montage. This implies that the potential is maximal at or near the location of the active electrode in the channel with the maximal deflection. As mentioned previously, referential montages are best suited for detecting broad

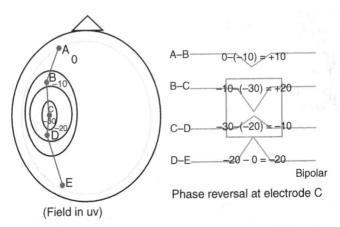

Figure 4.1 A phase reversal occurs between channels B–C and C–D as electrode C lies closest to the point of maximal potential (−30 uV).

or generalized potentials. They are limited by artifact and situations with an active reference (Chapter 5) [2]. Figure 4.2 explains the formation of maximal amplitude in a referential montage over a hypothetical potential.

Localization in Practice

A focal discharge is an epileptiform waveform that suggests the possible location of cortical irritability or tendency to generate seizures. Figure 4.3 shows a focal discharge on a longitudinal bipolar montage. There is a distinct phase reversal over the F4 electrode (channels Fp2-F4 and F4-C4). This location remains consistent when viewed in transverse montage (Figure 4.4). Furthermore, using an ipsilateral ear referential montage (Figure 4.5) shows that the discharge appears tallest (maximal amplitude) in the F4-A2 channel. Therefore, this potential focus resulting in the epileptic discharge localizes to the right frontal region (F4 electrode). As previously mentioned, this inference doesn't precisely correlate with the cortical anatomy (i.e., the right frontal lobe). It only estimates the general region where the focus of maximal potential generating the waveform of interest may originate.

Special Situations with Bipolar Montages

Isopotentials: If the maximal potential is large enough to involve two adjacent electrodes, then that channel will be neutral. There may be a phase reversal in

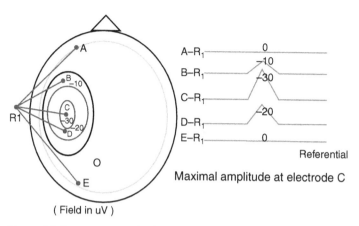

(Field in uV)

Figure 4.2 The same potential in Figure 4.1 on an ipsilateral ear referential montage. Electrode C lies closest to the point of maximal potential (−30 uV), therefore amplitude of deflection is greatest in channel C-R1.

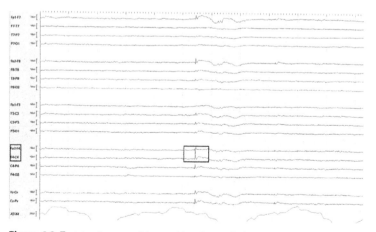

Figure 4.3 Twenty-nine-year-old man with epilepsy, discharge shows phase reversal at F4 (between channels Fp2-F4 and F4-C4) in longitudinal bipolar montage.

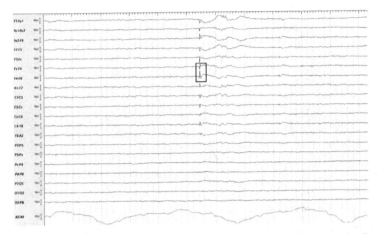

Figure 4.4 Same patient as in Figure 4.3, discharge again shows a phase reversal at F4 (between channels Fz-F4 and F4-F8) in transverse bipolar montage.

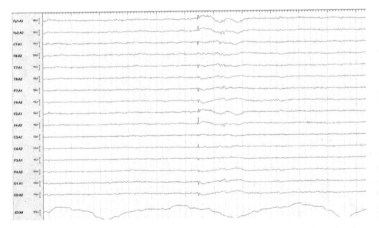

Figure 4.5 Same patient as in Figure 4.3, discharge again shows maximal amplitude at F4 (channel F4-A2) in ipsilateral ear (A2) referential montage.

the channels above and below the neutral channel. Therefore, phase reversals need not be adjacent to each other. However, nonadjacent phase reversals are separated by an isopotential channel (nearly flat line). Figure 4.6 shows T7-P7 at isopotential in a patient with left temporal discharges.

End of Chain Potential: If the maximal potential lies at or near the last electrode (end of chain) in a bipolar montage, such as O1 in a longitudinal bipolar montage, then there will be no phase reversal as there is no electrode to straddle the potential. The waveform generated by this potential will simply have maximal amplitude at the terminal electrode without a phase reversal. In these situations, the reader should use another bipolar montage perpendicular to the initial chain (such as a circumferential montage). A referential montage can also be used.

Phase Reversals on a Referential Montage

Phase reversals are the key to localization on bipolar montages but not referential montages except in two situations.

Horizontal Dipole: If the dipole lies horizontally (not radially as is typical) then both polar ends can be recorded off the scalp leading to a phase reversal on the referential montage. These are characteristically seen in benign epilepsy with centrotemporal spikes (described in Chapter 21).

Active Reference: If the reference is active due to contamination from an artifact potential, it may also lead to an apparent phase reversal at an electrode near another distant potential. Chapter 5 describes the active reference.

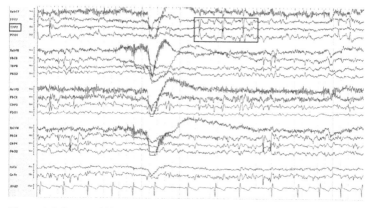

Figure 4.6 Six-year-old boy with cerebral palsy and multifocal epilepsy, left temporal discharges that show isopotential between T7 and P7.

Chapter Summary

1. Localization is the art of locating the site of maximal potential, presumably the origin of a waveform of interest.
2. The EEG is relatively blind to certain cortical regions, such as the sulcal depths, inferior surfaces of the brain, and infoldings such as the insula.
3. Localization depends on the montage in use and the rule of polarity.
4. Phase reversal is the key to localization with a bipolar montage. It is not diagnostic of an abnormality.
5. Maximal amplitude is the key to localization with a referential montage.
6. Phase reversals are usually but not always adjacent. Nonadjacent phase reversals are separated by an isopotential channel (near flat line).
7. Foci located at the end of a chain in a bipolar montage don't show a phase reversal.
8. An apparent phase reversal on a referential montage may indicate a horizontal dipole or an active reference.

References

1. Lagerlund TD. Manipulating the magic of digital EEG: montage reformatting and filtering. *American Journal of Electroneurodiagnostic Technology*. 2000 Jun 1;**40**(2):121–36.

2. Acharya JN, Acharya VJ. Overview of EEG montages and principles of localization. *Journal of Clinical Neurophysiology*. 2019 Sep 1;**36**(5):325–9.

Active Reference

A referential montage is only as good as its reference electrode.

The reference electrode is intended to be at a distant and neutral compared to the active electrode which lies close to the potential focus (maximal potential) of cerebral activity. However, if the potential focus lies at the reference electrode or if the reference is contaminated by artifactual potentials, then it becomes an active reference. Such a reference is no longer neutral and may mislead the reader into false localization.

There are two distinct possibilities the reader should consider when suspecting an active reference:

1. The reference lies at or near the potential focus.
2. The reference lies away from the potential focus but is contaminated by artifact.

When the reference is active because it is at or near the potential focus, all the channels in that referential montage will show deflections in the same direction. These may be of similar or different amplitudes but their deflections will all be in the same direction (waveforms will have the same polarities). In fact, those channels with the least amplitude lie closest to the focus (Figure 5.1).

The reference may also be active due to contamination by artifactual potentials. If a significant potential focus lies distant to the contaminated reference, an apparent phase reversal may occur at the channel closest to the focus. This is because both the contaminated reference electrode and the electrode close to the focus are active. As always, the direction of deflection at this channel will be governed by the law of polarity, that is, the pointer deflects toward the relatively negative electrode (Figure 5.2).

Each reference has its own common culprit artifact and no single reference is ideal for every situation. The choice of reference should be individualized based on the suspected location of the waveform and the contaminants common to that point of reference.

Central reference (Cz) is good for evaluating temporal waveforms but commonly contaminated by sleep potentials. Hence, Cz is best employed to evaluate temporal patterns during wakefulness. Ear references (such as

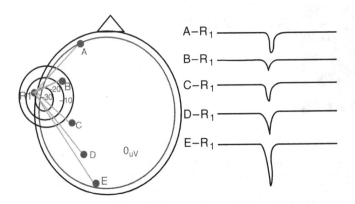

Potentials in microvolts (uV)

Figure 5.1 An active reference due to a hypothetical focus near the reference (R1); note the positive (downward) deflection in all channels. Channel B-R1 has the least deflection, as electrode B lies closest to the focus, while channel E-R1 has the largest deflection, as electrode E is most distant from the focus.

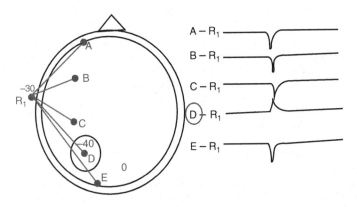

Potentials in microvolts (uV)

Figure 5.2 An active reference due to an artifactual potential (−30 uV) at R1. Additionally, there is a distant potential (−40 uV) at electrode D. Note the negative (upward) deflection in channel D-R1, as D is relatively more negative than R1. There are positive deflections (downward) in the other channels due to the negative contaminant potential at R1. This gives the appearance of a phase reversal on this ipsilateral ear referential montage.

ipsilateral and contralateral ear) are good for evaluation of central waveforms but they are commonly contaminated by EKG and temporalis muscle artifacts. Temporal discharges may also originate close to the ear reference. Therefore, ear references are best employed to evaluate central patterns during drowsiness or sleep. Similarly, a frontal reference (Fz) is good to evaluate an occipital pattern but commonly contaminated by eye movement artifact while occipital references (Oz) are good for frontal patterns but are contaminated by the posterior-dominant rhythm. If an active reference is detected, then an alternative referential montage should be used to confirm localization. Digital displays make switching between differential montages easy [1,2].

Chapter Summary

1. Referential montages are only as good as their reference electrode.
2. The reference electrode is intended to be distant from the potential focus and inactive, but sometimes it may be very active. This is called an active reference; it misleads the reader into false localization.
3. An active reference occurs if the reference electrode lies close to the potential focus or becomes contaminated by artifactual potentials.
4. If the reference is at or near the focus, typically there is a unidirectional reflection (often with varying amplitudes) in all the channels.
5. If the reference is contaminated by an artifactual potential, typically there is a phase reversal over channels that overlie a potential focus.
6. Central references are prone to contamination with sleep potentials, and ear references are prone to contamination with EKG and temporalis artifact.
7. Switch to an alternative referential montage if you suspect an active reference. This is easy with a digital display.

References

1. Teplan M. Fundamentals of EEG measurement. *Measurement Science Review.* 2002 Jan;2(2):1.

2. Lagerlund TD. Manipulating the magic of digital EEG: montage reformatting and filtering. *American Journal of Electroneurodiagnostic Technology.* 2000 Jun 1;40(2):121–36.

Chapter

6

Frequencies and Rhythms

As the initial step toward interpretation, the reader should clearly understand these two terms.

Frequency

Frequency is the number of times a waveform occurs per second (one big square). If a waveform occurs three times in a second, then its frequency is 3 Hz. If it occurs once over 2 s, then its frequency is 0.5 Hz. Therefore, the frequency simply describes the rate at which a waveform occurs, it doesn't indicate if that waveform is normal or abnormal. Conventionally, electroencephalographers group frequencies into standardized ranges (or bands) based on the Greek numeral.

They include delta, theta, alpha, beta, and gamma in increasing order of frequency (these exact cut offs may vary):

- Delta activity occurs with a frequency of 0.5 to 4 Hz.
- Theta activity occurs with a frequency of 5 to 7 Hz.
- Alpha activity occurs with a frequency of 8 to 13 Hz.
- Beta activity occurs with a frequency of 14 to 30 Hz.

Most electrographic activity on scalp EEG occurs between 0.5 to 30 Hz. The amplitude of the activity is usually inversely related to its frequency so lower frequencies typically have higher amplitudes compared to faster frequencies, but this isn't a rule.

Electrographic activities with frequencies above 30 Hz are called high-frequency oscillations (HFOs). These include gamma activity (30–80 Hz), ripples (80–200 Hz) and fast ripples (200–500 Hz). HFOs are difficult to appreciate on scalp EEG. Frequencies below 0.5 Hz are called infra-slow oscillations (IFOs) and are seen in preterm neonates [1].

Rhythm

A rhythm is a specific pattern of electrographic activity with a characteristic frequency. Therefore, in addition to frequency, rhythms have a typical location, morphology, and reactivity. Rhythms are also dependent on the physiological state such as wakefulness, drowsiness, or sleep (state dependence). Unlike frequency, rhythms indicate if the EEG is normal or abnormal. The reader should recognize the common rhythms and understand their implications [1].

As an example, alpha activity is not the same as an alpha rhythm. Any electrographic activity that occurs within the range of 8 to 13 Hz (alpha range) is termed *alpha activity*. However, the *alpha rhythm* specifically refers to the 8–13 Hz (alpha frequency) pattern with a posterior dominance (location) and sinusoidal appearance (morphology) that attenuates with eye opening (reactivity) that is seen during normal wakefulness (state dependence). Furthermore, alpha activity may be normal or abnormal, but alpha rhythm is the electrographic hallmark of normal wakefulness.

Alpha Rhythm

Recognizing the alpha rhythm is the starting point of all EEG interpretation. Historically, this was the first rhythm to be identified and it is thought to represent the resting activity of the occipital cortex. As mentioned in the previous example; during normal wakefulness, a posterior-predominant pattern of 8 to 13 Hz frequency (alpha frequency) occurs symmetrically over the occipital regions – this is the "normal" posterior-dominant rhythm (PDR). When this posterior-dominant rhythm attenuates with eye opening (reactivity) it is called the "alpha rhythm" – an obligate feature of normal adult wakefulness.

The posterior-dominant rhythm first attains a frequency of about 8 Hz at approximately 2–3 years of age will remain stable within the alpha range (commonly 9–10 Hz) till about the ninth decade of life, after which there may be a slight decline. The alpha rhythm is best appreciated in a relaxed state with eyes closed and attenuates with eye opening or intellectual effort. Figure 6.1 shows an 11 Hz alpha rhythm.

Normal Variations of the Alpha Rhythm

Alpha Squeak

This is a transient increase in the frequency of the alpha rhythm immediately after eye closure. Predigital era EEG machines had ink pens, these produced a squeaking noise each time the patient blinked, hence its name.

The reader must count the frequency of the posterior-dominant rhythm a second after eye closure to avoid overestimating it (avoid the squeak). Figure 6.1 shows the correct method to count the frequency of the posterior-dominant rhythm while Figure 6.2 shows prominent alpha squeak.

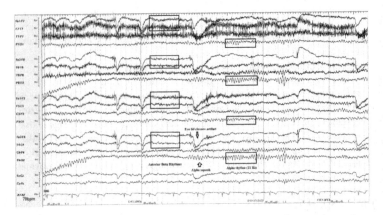

Figure 6.1 Twenty-seven-year-old woman with anxiety, anterior beta, and posterior alpha rhythms.

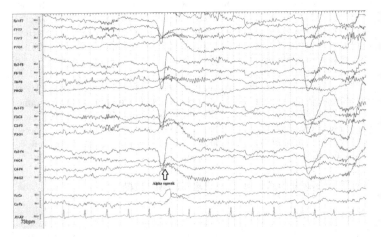

Figure 6.2 Thirty-four-year-old woman with starring spells, prominent alpha squeak.

Amplitude

The typical amplitude (voltage) of the alpha rhythm is 30–40 uV, but there is considerable variation. Lower amplitudes may result in poor visualization of the alpha rhythm in as many as a quarter of normal adults. In these circumstances, the sensitivity may be increased.

Symmetry

A slight asymmetry of alpha amplitude and frequency between the two hemispheres is normal. The dominant hemisphere (commonly left) may have a slightly lower amplitude compared to the nondominant side (commonly right).

Paradoxical Alpha

Normally, the alpha rhythm attenuates with eye opening. Sometimes during drowsiness, it may paradoxically increase with eye opening – paradoxical alpha.

Slow and Fast Alpha Variants

Alpha variants include slow and fast variants that show a harmonic relationship but with similar distribution and reactivity. Slow variants have frequencies typically half that of alpha (4–5 Hz) and fast variants have frequencies twice that of alpha (16–20 Hz). Occasionally, these variants may have a notched appearance [2]. Figure 6.3 shows a slow alpha variant.

Abnormalities of the Alpha Rhythm

The alpha rhythm may be abnormal if it is slow, asymmetric or unreactive (Bancaud's phenomena).

Generalized Slowing: This occurs if the alpha rhythm does not exceed 8 Hz at any point during the recording. Though 8 Hz is the lower normal of alpha range, this frequency is thought to occur in less than 1% of normal adults. Figure 6.4 shows generalized slowing.

Asymmetry: Amplitude asymmetry of greater than 50% is abnormal especially if the dominant hemisphere (commonly left) is greater than the nondominant hemisphere (commonly right). Normally, the frequency between hemispheres differs by less than 0.5–1 Hz. Asymmetries of more than 1 Hz are abnormal.

Bancaud's Phenomenon: This refers to the failure of the alpha rhythm to attenuate with eye opening on the side ipsilateral to a structural abnormality. This is usually associated with occipital or pontine lesions [2].

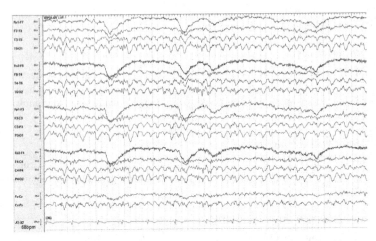

Figure 6.3 Twenty-seven-year-old man with syncope, slow alpha variant (4 Hz).

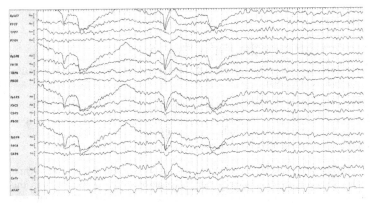

Figure 6.4 Seventy-two-year-old woman with dementia, mild generalized alpha slowing (8 Hz).

Beta Rhythm

Beta rhythms have frequencies of 14 Hz or greater (commonly 18–25 Hz). They have a low amplitude (less than 20 uV) and an anterior predominance.

Beta rhythms are thought to represent the resting activity of the precentral cortex; they tend to attenuate with contralateral movements (much like the "mu" rhythm which is described later in Chapter 13). Normally, beta rhythms occur during wakefulness and accentuate during drowsiness and light sleep. Speech and intellectual efforts also accentuate beta rhythms. Figure 6.1 shows the normal anterior beta rhythm during wakefulness.

Excessive Beta

This is usually the result of sedatives such as benzodiazepines and barbiturates. There may be increased amplitude (>25 uV), prevalence (>50% of the record) and/or generalized distribution of beta rhythm. Figure 6.5 shows excessive beta associated with benzodiazepine use.

Asymmetric Beta

The persistent suppression of beta over a region or hemisphere may indicate an ipsilateral cortical abnormality or an interruption between the cortical surface and the recording electrode such as a subdural hematoma or scalp edema. Conversely, breach effect may result in an increase in beta amplitudes due to loss of skull bone [2].

Theta Rhythm

Theta rhythms have frequencies of 5 to 7 Hz with varying amplitudes and morphology. A third of teens and young adults normally have 6 to 7 Hz theta over the frontocentral region during wakefulness. This may be enhanced with

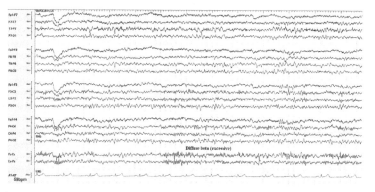

Figure 6.5 Fifty-six-year-old woman with epilepsy on clobazam, diffuse beta rhythms (excessive beta).

emotions, focused concentration, or mental tasks. Also, a third of asymptomatic elderly will have intermittent 5–6 Hz theta over the bitemporal regions (usually left greater than right).

However, in most normal adults, theta rhythms are limited to drowsiness or light sleep and their presence during wakefulness is abnormal [2]. Midline theta may occur as a normal variant as described in Chapter 13.

Delta Rhythm

Delta rhythms have frequencies below 4 Hz. In young children, their prevalence normally doesn't exceed 10% of the waking record and in the elderly, rare intrusions of isolated delta (often over the left temporal region) during drowsiness may be permissible.

However, in most normal adults, delta rhythms are limited to sleep and their presence during wakefulness is abnormal. Focal delta may indicate underlying cerebral lesions and diffuse delta may indicate generalized cerebral dysfunction or encephalopathy [2]. Figure 6.6 shows theta and delta rhythms in encephalopathy.

Chapter Summary

1. Frequency is the number of times a waveform occurs per second (one big square).
2. Rhythms in addition to frequency have characteristic features of location, morphology, reactivity, and state dependence.
3. Frequencies are descriptive; rhythms are diagnostic.

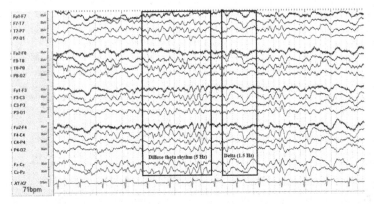

Figure 6.6 Sixty-two-year-old man with hepatic failure, diffuse theta and delta rhythms.

4. Clinically relevant frequency bands include delta (0.5–4 Hz), theta (5–7 Hz), alpha (8–13 Hz), and beta (14–30 Hz).
5. The alpha rhythm is an obligate feature of normal wakefulness; it has considerable variations.
6. Abnormal alpha rhythm may be slow, asymmetric, or unreactive (Bancaud's phenomena).
7. Excessive beta is associated with sedative medications.
8. In most normal adults, theta and delta rhythms are limited to drowsiness or sleep; their occurrence during wakefulness may be abnormal.

References

1. Nayak CS, Anilkumar AC. EEG normal waveforms. *InStatPearls* [Internet] 2020 Jun 28.

2. Tatum WO IV, Husain AM, Benbadis SR, Kaplan PW. Normal adult EEG and patterns of uncertain significance. *Journal of Clinical Neurophysiology*. 2006 Jun 1;**23**(3):194–207.

Chapter 7

Maturation

Electrographic activity undergoes serial change from birth through the pediatric age group into adulthood. Interpreting the developing EEG is challenging, but the basic principles of EEG interpretation remain the same for all ages. Neonatal and infantile studies require special accommodations for recording and review. The EEGs of older children and adolescents resemble those of adults. Interpreting neonatal EEGs, especially those of prematurity, requires a level of expertise beyond the scope of most trainees. They will not be discussed here in detail. This chapter is intended as an introductory framework on maturation rather than as a reference for neonatal EEG interpretations, for which the reader is directed to a standard textbook on the subject.

Recording EEGs in Children

The reader should be familiar with a few important aspects of recording EEGs in early life.

Placement

Neonates often require a reduced electrode array due to a smaller head size. At a minimum, Fp1/2, C3/Cz/C4, T7/8, O1/2, and ear lobes (A1/2) or mastoids (M1/2) should be used. Cz (midline) is recommended in neonates, as positive sharp waves typically occur in this channel. The head size in children increases until about 3 years, allowing more electrodes to be added. Older children may be recorded with a full set of electrodes [1].

Parameters

The American Society of Clinical Neurophysiology (ACNS) recommends using a sensitivity of 7 uV/mm and a low-frequency filter between 0.3 and 0.6 Hz (time contrast 0.27–0.53 s) for neonatal records. The adult setting of 1 Hz (time constant 0.16 s) is inadequate for low-voltage fast activities. Children have higher background voltages than adults, so sensitivity may be reduced to 10 or 15 uV/mm as appropriate. The standard paper speed is 30 mm/s, but neonatal records are often compressed to 15 mm/s, resulting in a sharper appearance [1,2].

Polygraphy

The sleep–wake cycle is poorly differentiated in neonates. Additional noncerebral parameters called polygraphs are needed to help differentiate physiological states. Polygraphs are also useful for characterizing physiological artifacts and symptoms such as apnea or arrythmia. Standard polygraphs include respiration, heart rate (EKG), eye movements (EOG), and muscle movements (Chin EMG). Synchronous video allows event characterization. Additional measures, such as upper airway exchange and oxygen saturation, are needed in infants with apneic events [1].

Sleep

Efforts should be made to include sleep, as it helps interpret cerebral maturation. Epileptic discharges also accentuate during light sleep. In children, the sleep record is easier to interpret compared to wakefulness as there is less movement artifact. Feeding or sleep deprivation will improve the chances of recording sleep. Sedatives are discouraged, but oral melatonin may occasionally be useful. Standard recordings should be of at least 1 hour duration to obtain a complete sleep cycle [1]. Figure 7.1 shows a typical neonatal recording with polygraphs.

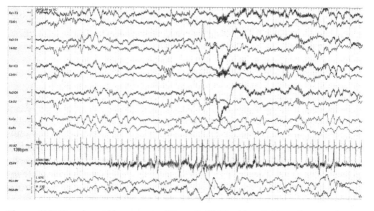

Figure 7.1 Two-day-old boy at term (39 weeks PMA) with twitching, showing the typical channels of a neonatal record (sensitivity 15 uV).

Basics of Interpretation

The EEG in neonates should be interpreted in the context of two key reference points. These are postmenstrual age (PMA) and physiological state (awake or asleep). These determine the normal expectations for electrographic activity. Persistent deviations outside of these expectations indicate dysmaturity and consequently a greater risk of abnormal neurological outcomes. The sleep–wake cycle and age-specific electrographic patterns (graphoelements) provide additional information about maturity.

Postmenstrual Age (PMA)

Postmenstrual age is the sum of gestational age at birth (number of weeks from the first day of last menstrual period) and chronological age at time of recording (number of weeks postpartum). *Term* is defined as 37–44 weeks PMA, while less than 37 weeks is *preterm* and 44–48 weeks is *postterm*. Traditionally, conceptual age (CA) has also been used. The CA is shorter than the PMA, as the last menstrual period occurs about two weeks before conception [3].

The normal adult EEG is a culmination of serial age-dependent changes of maturation. Assuming other parameters remain constant, there aren't significant differences in the appearance of EEGs among healthy infants of similar PMA, even though gestational ages may differ. For example, the EEG of a healthy 4-week-old baby born at 36 weeks gestation (PMA 40 weeks) is similar to that of a 2-week-old baby born at 38 weeks gestation (PMA also 40 weeks). Premature births will lack the features of a term birth, but these eventually catch up with time. Initially, appreciable changes occur every two to four weeks, but later, the pace slows. By early childhood (1–3 years), the record begins to resemble adulthood and reaches near-maturity in preschool children (3–5 years), with a few minor transformations thereafter [3,4].

Physiological State (Wakefulness, Active, or Quiet Sleep)

EEGs must be interpreted in the context of physiological state (wakefulness or sleep). This is easier in older children and adults but challenging in neonates, as specific sleep architecture is not developed. As the EEG alone isn't enough to determine state, the reader must rely on polygraphs and observation (bedside or video). A clear physiological state typically lasts for at least a minute. The reader must evaluate if the electrographic features during this time are consistent with those normally expected for that state in the context of the PMA. Wakefulness is characterized by open eyes, and this remains the sole identifying feature before 30 weeks PMA, after which polygraphs including respiration and EMG activity become useful. The awake neonate may be active (movements) or quiet (wide-open eyes but not moving). Sleep is classified as active (precursor of rapid eye movement [REM] sleep) and quiet sleep (precursor of slow-wave sleep). The normal sleep–wake cycle itself changes through infancy and childhood, as described below [4].

Principles of Maturation

The reader must estimate if the EEG lies within the normal limits of maturation within the context of the PMA and physiological state. This evaluation is based on the predominant electrographic activity (also called background), the sleep–wake cycle, and graphoelements. Continuity and synchrony form the key components of the background development. As the brain matures, the EEG becomes progressively more continuous and synchronous, along with other features, such as voltage, variability, and reactivity. The sleep–wake cycle begins to resemble adults', and transitional graphoelements disappear.

Continuity

Continuity refers to continuous or uninterrupted electrographic activity. Discontinuous periods have a voltage less than 25 uV (attenuation). In a continuous record, these should not exceed 2 s in duration. Sustained continuity is the hallmark of maturation, while persistent discontinuity indicates dysmaturity. The normal neonatal EEG is discontinuous (*trace discontinu*) irrespective of physiological state before 30 weeks PMA. Thereafter, the record becomes progressively more continuous during wakefulness and active sleep (trace discontinu becomes restricted to quiet sleep). At term, the normal neonatal EEG is nearly continuous in all states including quiet sleep. The EEG in a healthy term neonate in quiet sleep shows a continuous but alternating pattern (trace alternans); this is the mature form of trace discontinu. Trace alternans is replaced by slow waves around 42–46 weeks (slow-wave sleep). Figure 7.2 shows persistent discontinuity (dysmaturity) in a term neonate [3].

Synchrony

The near-simultaneous onset of electrographic activity in both hemispheres is called synchrony. Minor lags are permissible (within 1.5 s), but to be synchronous, the overall majority of electrographic activity should begin simultaneously in both hemispheres. The neonatal EEG is normally synchronous before 30 weeks PMA but becomes asynchronous between 30 and 37 weeks, after which synchrony is again restored. As the normal neonatal EEG is synchronous by term, persistent asynchrony is abnormal [3].

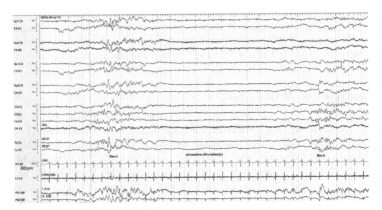

Figure 7.2 Four-day-old girl at term (39 weeks PMA) with neonatal seizures showing an abnormal pattern of persistent discontinuity (sensitivity 15 uV).

Voltage

Voltage is the amplitude or height of the electrographic activity. There is no consensus on the normal limits of voltage in prematurity, but healthy term neonates have voltage greater than 25 uV in all physiological states. Attenuation refers to voltages between 25 and 10 uV, while suppression refers to those less than 10 uV. Suppression suggests severe neuronal dysfunction or injury. The absence of electrographic activity of more than 2 uV when reviewed at a sensitivity of 2 uV/mm is called electrocerebral inactivity (ECI). Several extracerebral conditions, such as poor electrode placement, scalp swelling, and subdural hemorrhage, may also artificially reduce the voltage [3].

Variability and Reactivity

Variability refers to spontaneous changes in the electrographic activity, such as those occurring with state changes (sleep–wake cycle). These normally become established at 30 weeks PMA. Reactivity refers to changes in the electrographic activity occurring secondary to an external stimulus. These may be elicited from around 32 weeks PMA [3]. Both variability and reactivity are discussed in greater detail in Chapter 10.

Maturation of the Sleep–Wake Cycle

Preterm neonates show the early signs of sleep–wake cycling prior to 30 weeks PMA. Later, around 40% of sleep is active, 30% is quiet, and 30% is indeterminate, with a duration of sleep cycle around 30–50 min until term. Healthy term neonates normally have a complete sleep–wake cycle over 3 hours and a sleep-only cycle (active–transition–quiet) over an hour. For the first 3 months of age, the infant first falls into active sleep (precursor of REM sleep); later, the infant falls into quiet sleep (precursor of slow-wave sleep) and then transitions to active sleep like adults. Early portions of the EEG during quiet sleep may show trace alternans, but this is replaced with continuous high-voltage slow waves (slow-wave sleep) with maturity. At term, about 50% of sleep is active, whereas in adults, about 20% is REM sleep. The duration of each stage of sleep is about 20 min, though it may be longer. Therefore, standard recordings should be at least 1 hour in duration to obtain a complete sleep cycle [3].

Graphoelements

Graphoelements are distinct neonatal waveforms that temporarily appear during development in an age-dependent manner. These patterns are embedded into the electrographic activity. They appear during specific ranges of PMA and then disappear. Early examples of graphoelements include monorhythmic delta, delta brushes, and rhythmic temporal delta activity. Anterior dysthymia and enconches fontanelles typically occur between 32 and 44 weeks PMA. Anterior dysrhythmia consists of symmetric and synchronous delta runs over the frontal region. Enconches fontanelles are broad-pointed diphasic waves with a small initial upward (negative) deflection followed by a large downward (positive) deflection, most prevalent in transitional sleep. Figure 7.3 shows anterior dysrhythmia and enconches fontanelles [3,4].

EEG of Neonates and Preterm Births

Wakefulness

Wakefulness in a healthy term neonate is characterized by wide-open eyes and irregular respirations. Spontaneous limb and body movements may also occur. The corresponding EEG consists of continuous, medium-voltage (25–50 uV) theta and delta with overriding beta activities. This is called *activite moyenne* (French for "medium"). In premature neonates, prior to 30 weeks PMA, the record is normally discontinuous (trace discontinu). Brief portions of the waking record become continuous after 30 weeks PMA. The normal neonatal EEG is nearly continuous during wakefulness by 34 weeks PMA to term [3]. Figure 7.3 shows the normal EEG of wakefulness at term.

Sleep

Neonatal sleep may be active (precursor of REM sleep) or quiet (precursor of slow-wave sleep). Additionally, transitional and indeterminate stages occur.

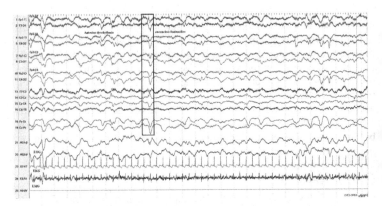

Figure 7.3 Nine-day-old boy at term (40 weeks PMA) during wakefulness showing activite moyenne along with anterior dysrhythmia and enconches fontanelles (sensitivity 15 uV).

During the first 3 months of life, the neonate first falls into active sleep and then transitions to quiet sleep, followed again by active sleep. Later, drowsiness is followed by quiet and then active sleep. This pattern continues in later life, when slow-wave sleep is followed by REM sleep.

Active Sleep
Healthy term neonates in active sleep have their eyes closed, intermittent periods of REM, axial muscular atonia, twitching or jerking movements (myoclonus), and irregular respirations and heart rate. The EEG background shows *activite moyenne*, like that of normal wakefulness. In preterm births prior to 30 weeks PMA, the record in active sleep is discontinuous (trace discontinu), but by 30 weeks, the typical features of active sleep, such as REM, irregular respirations, and body movements, emerge, along with a more continuous EEG. After 34 weeks PMA to term, active sleep in the preterm nearly resembles that of a term neonate with continuous EEG background (activite moyenne). Figure 7.4 shows the normal EEG of active sleep at term.

Quiet Sleep
Healthy term neonates in quiet sleep have their eyes closed, with regular respirations and heart rate. Their movements are minimal (occasional sucking or startles), and rapid eye movements are absent. The EEG background may shows *trace alternans* characterized by alternations of higher voltage at 4- to 5-s bursts (50–150 uV) and brief, low-voltage (25–50 uV) interburst intervals.

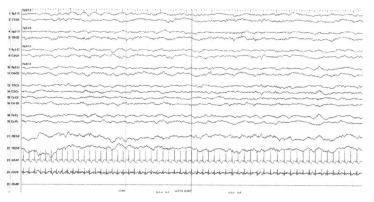

Figure 7.4 Same patient as in Figure 7.3 in active sleep, also showing activite moyenne (sensitivity 15 uV).

The bursts are composed of delta slowing, while there is mixed theta and delta activity during the interburst interval (like activite moyenne). This pattern begins to fade around 42 weeks and disappears by 46 weeks. At this time, quiet sleep is characterized by a continuous higher-voltage, mixed delta and theta background (slow waves). Early sleep spindles (10–12 Hz) first appear at 46 weeks PMA. In preterm neonates, the record is discontinuous irrespective of state prior to 30 weeks PMA. Later, the record becomes progressively more continuous during wakefulness and active sleep but remains discontinuous (trace discontinu) during quiet sleep. Trace discontinu matures into trace alternans at term. Figure 7.5 shows the normal EEG of quiet sleep at term.

Transitional Sleep and Indeterminate Sleep

Temporary stages of incomplete sleep occurring between wakefulness and active and quiet sleep are called transitional sleep. In preterm (especially before 30 weeks), most sleep cannot be properly distinguished into active and quiet sleep, so this is called indeterminate sleep. With an increase in PMA, the periods of indeterminate sleep become limited to transitions between physiological states (transitional sleep) and minimum near term (10%–15%). Excessive amounts of indeterminate sleep in a term neonate may be a sign of abnormality [3].

EEG of Infancy

The EEG in early infancy (first 3 months) is characterized by fading away of neonatal patterns, which are replaced by patterns resembling the electrographic activity of adulthood.

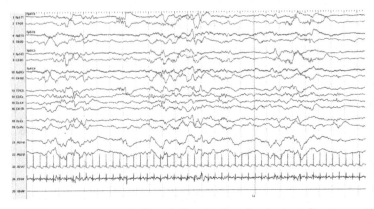

Figure 7.5 Same patient as in Figure 7.3 in quiet sleep, showing trace alternans (sensitivity 15 uV).

Wakefulness

The background frequency begins to transition from the upper delta range (3–4 Hz) to the lower theta range (5–6 Hz) at 3–5 months of age and reaches up to 7 Hz at the end of the first year. Gradually, the emerging posterior-dominant rhythm shows reactivity to eye blink at 3–4 months. Figure 7.6 shows normal EEG of wakefulness in an infant.

Drowsiness

Drowsiness (transition from wakefulness to sleep) is typically characterized by slowing of the electrographic activity to delta range (3–4 Hz). Hypersynchrony refers to generalized bursts of rhythmic, high-amplitude delta (about 4 Hz) that occur during state changes in late infancy (3–12 months) and childhood but sometimes persist in young adults. When hypersynchrony occurs during transition to sleep (drowsiness), it is called hypnogogic hypersynchrony, and when it occurs during arousal from sleep, it is called hypnopompic hypersynchrony. Hypersynchronous bursts may be misidentified as generalized spike wave discharges, especially when faster frequencies are superimposed. However, on close review, the spikes will not be truly associated with after-coming slow waves (more on these later in Chapter 14) [3]. Drowsiness can be easily identified electrographically during transitions after 9 months of age.

Sleep

The trace alternans pattern of neonatal quiet sleep transitions to an occipital-predominant, high-amplitude (150–200 uV), diffuse, polymorphic delta

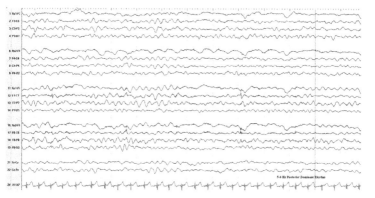

Figure 7.6 Nine-month-old boy with hiccups, 5–6 Hz posterior-dominant rhythm during wakefulness (sensitivity 20 uV). A posterior-dominant rhythm first appears at three months of age.

activity by 42–46 weeks PMA (slow-wave sleep). Asynchronous sleep spindles (12–15 Hz) become apparent over the central regions before 3 months and synchronize after 6 months of age. REM sleep is electrographically characterized by eye movement artifact and diffuse high-voltage delta or theta activities similar to wakefulness. Figure 7.7 shows synchronous sleep spindles.

Sleep–Wake Cycle

The time spent in REM sleep decreases with increasing maturity. It is around 50% at birth and falls to around 40% at 4 months and then 30% after the first year. It is about 20% in adults [4].

EEG of Early Childhood (1–5 Years)

The posterior-dominant rhythm (PDR) attains alpha range (8 Hz) around 2–3 years of age, with some variability. Hypersynchronous bursts decrease in occurrence by around 3 years of age. Drowsiness in children may be heralded by bursts of frontal-predominant theta activity. Stage II (spindle sleep) is now distinctly characterized by synchronous sleep spindles along with prominent vertex waves and K complexes. Stage III (slow-wave sleep) is characterized by posterior-predominant diffuse delta waves, and REM sleep shows diffuse medium-amplitude theta activities. During the preschool years (ages 3–5 years), the normal posterior-dominant rhythm is alpha, though some intermixed theta frequencies are common. Hypnogogic hypersynchrony usually disappears after the age of 3 years. Slow-wave sleep in this age group shows

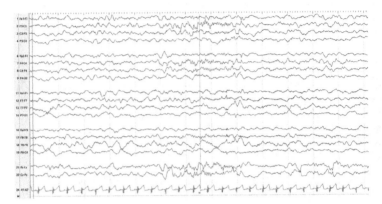

Figure 7.7 Same patient as in Figure 7.6 showing synchronous sleep spindles (sensitivity 20 uV). Asynchronous sleep spindles first appear before three months of age and synchronize around six months of age.

diffuse slow waves with less of an occipital predominance compared to younger children, and REM sleep shows a low-voltage theta background. Preschool children may also cooperate with activation procedures, such as hyperventilation and photic stimulation [4].

EEG of Late Childhood and Adolescence (6–18 Years)

After around 10 years of age, the normal posterior-dominant rhythm during wakefulness is around 10 Hz. Posterior slow waves of youth are common at this age. Hypnogogic hypersynchrony is rarely seen after 6 years of age. A prominent hyperventilation response is common in this age group. Maturation slows during this period, as the EEG closely resembles adulthood [4]. Figure 7.8 shows hypersynchrony during arousal.

Chapter Summary

1. Neonatal EEGs should be interpreted in the context of postmenstrual age (PMA) and physiological state (awake, active, or quite sleep).
2. Sustained continuity is the hallmark of maturation. Early preterm records are discontinuous (trace discontinu) irrespective of state, whereas term records are near-continuous in all states. Between 30 and 37 weeks, the record becomes more continuous during wakefulness and active sleep, but it remains discontinuous during quiet sleep.

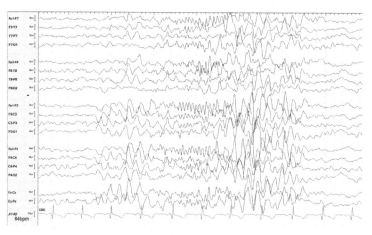

Figure 7.8 Nine-year-old boy with agitation shows hypersynchrony during an arousal (sensitivity 10 uV). Hypersynchrony first appears around three months of age and usually disappears by 3 years of age, though in some children, it may persist into adolescence.

3. Activite moyenne (continuous) is seen during wakefulness and active sleep in a healthy term neonate.

4. Trace alternans is seen during quiet sleep in a healthy term neonate.

5. At term, about 50% of sleep is active, whereas in adults, about 20% is REM sleep.

6. Anterior dysrhythmia and enconches fontanelles are common graphoelements that occur between 32 and 44 weeks PMA.

7. A reactive posterior-dominant rhythm emerges after 3 months of age.

8. Asynchronous sleep spindles appear before 3 months and synchronize by 6 months.

9. The posterior-dominant rhythm attains alpha range by 2–3 years of age.

10. Hypersynchrony appears around 3 months and resolves by 3 years; rarely, it may persist longer. It may be misidentified as generalized spike wave complexes.

References

1. Kuratani J, Pearl PL, Sullivan LR, et al. American Clinical Neurophysiology Society guideline 5: minimum technical standards for pediatric electroencephalography. *The Neurodiagnostic Journal*. 2016 Oct 1;**56**(4):266–75.

2. Britton JW, Frey LC, Hopp JL, et al. *Electroencephalography (EEG): an introductory text and atlas of normal and abnormal findings in adults, children, and infants*. American Epilepsy Society, Chicago; 2016.

3. Tsuchida TN, Wusthoff CJ, Shellhaas RA, et al. American clinical neurophysiology society standardized EEG terminology and categorization for the description of continuous EEG monitoring in neonates: report of the American Clinical Neurophysiology Society Critical Care Monitoring Committee. *Journal of Clinical Neurophysiology.* 2013 Apr 1;**30**(2):161–73.

4. Eisermann M, Kaminska A, Moutard ML, Soufflet C, Plouin P. Normal EEG in childhood: from neonates to adolescents. *Neurophysiologie clinique/Clinical Neurophysiology.* 2013 Jan 1;**43**(1):35–65.

Normal Adult EEG

The EEG normally remains relatively stable throughout adulthood, but it should be interpreted within the context of the physiological state. This chapter describes the normal EEG of adults during wakefulness, drowsiness, and sleep.

Wakefulness

In an awake resting adult, the normal EEG is characterized by a reactive, posterior-dominant alpha rhythm, usually in the range of 9–12 Hz with considerable individual variations. There is an anterior-predominant beta rhythm and admixtures of alpha and beta in the intermediate channels. Eye blink and muscle artifacts are present.

Additionally, certain normal variants such as lambda waves, posterior slow waves of youth and wicket waves may occur [1]. They are described in Chapter 13. Figure 8.1 shows a normal EEG during wakefulness.

Drowsiness

The typical transition to drowsiness is characterized by a decrease in the amplitude (attenuation) and slowing of the posterior-dominant alpha to theta temporally and occipitally. This change is especially prominent in the elderly. The anterior-predominant beta also increases in amplitude and slows to theta range, this leads to the emergence of diffuse theta (especially prominent in young adults). Slow lateral eye movements appear and muscle artifact dissipates. Figure 8.2 shows the normal EEG during drowsiness. Sometimes there may be a sudden symmetric sub-harmonic drop in frequency of the posterior-dominant rhythm (such as 10 Hz to 5 Hz). The point of the drop may resemble a sharp notch that can be mistaken for an abnormality. In others, the alpha may become paradoxically prominent with eye opening (paradoxical alpha). Rarely, beta enhancement also occurs [2]. Hypersynchrony may occur in young adults as described in Chapter 7.

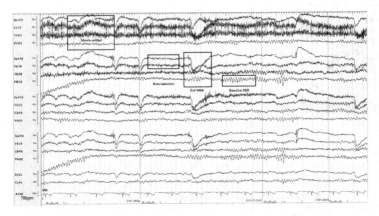

Figure 8.1 Twenty-three-year-old man with epilepsy, normal wakefulness characterized by a reactive posterior-dominant rhythm (11 Hz), low-amplitude frontal beta activity, eye blink, and temporalis muscle artifact.

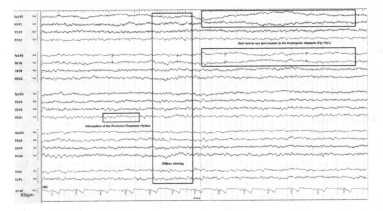

Figure 8.2 Same patient as in Figure 8.1, normal drowsiness characterized by attenuation of the posterior-dominant rhythm, emergence of theta range slowing and slow lateral eye movements. Note that the muscle artifact has dissipated.

Sleep

Normal sleep consists of non–rapid eye movement (NREM) and rapid eye movement (REM) sleep. Non–rapid eye movement sleep is further classified into stages I, II, and III (slow-wave sleep).

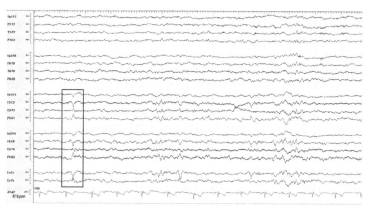

Figure 8.3 Same patient as in Figure 8.1, stage I sleep with vertex waves and POSTS.

Stage I (N1) sleep is marked by the appearance of vertex waves in the backdrop of drowsiness.

Vertex waves are centrally predominant (vertex), sharp transients (200 ms or more in duration) with maximal negativity at the Cz channel. They are characteristically bilateral, symmetric, and synchronous without an aftercoming slow wave. They may be induced by a sudden noise and abolished by arousal. In childhood and youth, they may have a prominent and sharper appearance but unlike central spikes (abnormality), vertex waves are state dependent and not consistently lateralized. Figure 8.3 shows vertex waves during stage I sleep.

Positive occipital sharp transients of sleep (POSTS) may also occur. These are described in Chapter 13.

Stage II (N2) sleep is marked by the appearance of sleep spindles and K complexes. They appear as cerebral activity progressively slows into theta and later delta range.

Sleep spindles are transient, frontocentral-predominant bursts of sinusoidal 10–14 Hz activity. They are normally symmetric and synchronous with maximal amplitude in the middle and tapering ends (spindle form).

K complex is a high-amplitude, central-predominant, diphasic complex with an initial sharp transient followed by a large slow wave with an associated sleep spindle that is best appreciated in the frontocentral region. K complexes may be induced by a loud noise. Persistent asymmetries of spindles and K complexes are suggestive of cerebral pathology ipsilateral to the side of their absence or attenuation. Figure 8.4 shows sleep spindles and K complexes during stage II sleep.

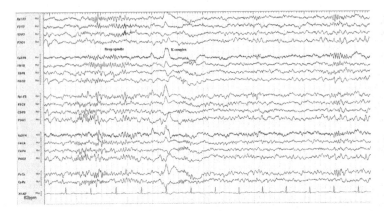

Figure 8.4 Same patient as in Figure 8.1, stage II sleep with sleep spindles and K complexes.

Sometimes, a sharper waveform may occur on the upslope of the slow wave of same polarity. This resembles the outline of a hand mitten with the "thumb" formed by the last wave of the spindle and the "hand" formed by the slow wave. These *mitten waves* are normal variants of the K complex. They have a frontocentral predominance and parasagittal spread. They are best appreciated on a referential montage. Figure 8.5 shows mitten waves. Rarely, epileptic discharges may be associated with K complexes as shown in Figure 8.6 – this is called dyshormia [3]. Epileptic discharges are described later in this book.

Stage III (N3 slow-wave sleep) is characterized by the emergence of higher amplitude (>75 uV), diffuse, 1–2 Hz semirhythmic delta slowing. Vertex waves, spindles, and K complexes persist during this stage. Figure 8.7 shows slow-wave sleep.

Rapid eye movement (REM sleep) is characterized by rapid eye movements, hypotonia (absence of muscle artifact) and sawtooth waves on the EEG. The background shows range slowing without any muscle artifact (like drowsiness). Rapid eye movements manifest as quick saccades in the frontopolar channels unlike the slow eye movements of drowsiness. Central sawtooth waves appear as rhythmic slowing in the central and parietal channels best seen on a referential montage. Figure 8.8 shows REM sleep. Most normal adults will spend 75% of their sleep in NREM and 25% in REM, these alternate in cycles four to six times in a normal night's sleep, each cycle about 90–110 min in duration. There is usually a predominance of NREM in the first part of the night and REM in the later third. Occasionally, a routine EEG may capture REM – this is usually from sleep deprivation and doesn't necessarily imply a diagnosis of narcolepsy [4].

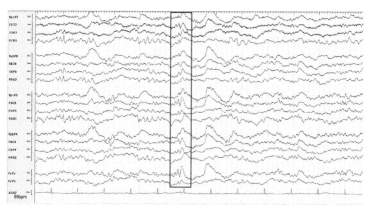

Figure 8.5 Same patient as in Figure 8.1, mitten waves.

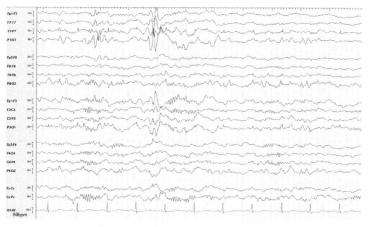

Figure 8.6 Fifty-two-year-old woman with mesial temporal lobe epilepsy, left temporal discharges associated with K complexes (dyshormia).

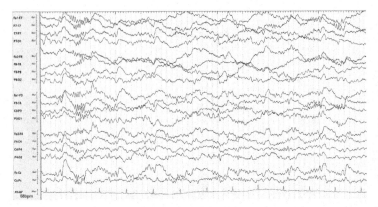

Figure 8.7 Sixty-two-year-old man with epilepsy, slow-wave sleep characterized by diffuse, high-amplitude, semirhythmic delta slowing.

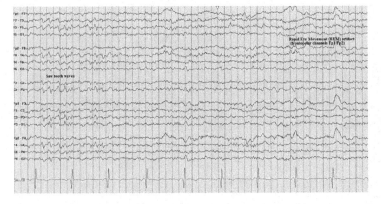

Figure 8.8 Thirty-two-year-old man with nocturnal movements, rapid eye movement artifact, and sawtooth waves during REM sleep.

Chapter Summary

1. The normal EEG doesn't change much during adult life, but it must be interpreted in the context of physiological states (awake, drowsy, or asleep).
2. Normal wakefulness is characterized by a reactive posterior-dominant alpha rhythm, anterior faster beta activity, eye blink, and muscle artifact.
3. Transition to drowsiness is typically characterized by attenuation of the posterior-dominant rhythm, diffuse slowing into theta range, emergence of slow lateral eye movements, and dissipation of muscle artifact.
4. Vertex waves are the architectural feature of stage I sleep. Positive occipital sharp transients of sleep (POSTS) may also occur.
5. Sleep spindles and K complexes are the architectural feature of stage II sleep.
6. Mitten waves are a normal variant, while dyshormia is abnormal.
7. Slow-wave sleep is characterized by diffuse high-amplitude semirhythmic delta slowing.
8. Rapid eye movement sleep is characterized by eye movement artifact and sawtooth waves.

References

1. Tatum WO IV, Husain AM, Benbadis SR, Kaplan PW. Normal adult EEG and patterns of uncertain significance. *Journal of Clinical Neurophysiology.* 2006 Jun 1;**23**(3):194–207.

2. Nayak CS, Anilkumar AC. *EEG normal waveforms.* InStatPearls [Internet] 2020 Jun 28.

3. Villamar MF, Gilliam FG. Dyshormia in focal epilepsy. *Arquivos de neuro-psiquiatria.* 2018 Jul;**76**(7):495–6.

4. Eisermann M, Kaminska A, Moutard ML, Soufflet C, Plouin P. Normal EEG in childhood: from neonates to adolescents. *Neurophysiologie clinique/Clinical Neurophysiology.* 2013 Jan 1;**43**(1):35–65.

Chapter **Approach to EEG Reading**

Let's start. I recommend this stepwise approach. The first step is the same as with any test, confirm the *patient's identity*. Be sure the EEG you are about to read belongs to the correct patient. Additionally, note three important points before reading. The technologist will usually mark these out for the reader.

1. *Age:* The EEG is relatively stable during adulthood. However, certain normal variants are common in young adults. A slight slowing of the posterior-dominant rhythm may be considered within normal after the age of 80, but it must remain within alpha range.
2. *State(s):* The EEG varies with state changes; it is important to note if the patient was awake, drowsy, or asleep during the record. Furthermore, epileptic discharges are accentuated during drowsiness and sleep. If the patient is confused or comatose, then the EEG is reflective of that state. More on this later.
3. *Skull defect:* The skull serves as a natural filter of higher frequencies. EEG activity over a skull defect such as a craniotomy is typically sharper, faster, and of higher amplitude compared to the rest of the skull. This is called a breach effect. *To avoid overcall, the sharpness of a waveform must be interpreted with caution over a skull defect* [1]. Most epileptic discharges are negative (upward) but with the alteration of neuronal dipoles from brain surgery, such as a temporal lobectomy, the discharges may be positive (downward) [2].

Next, open to view the record.

Before interpreting the EEG activity, *check the settings*. These are usually placed on the top in most digital displays. They include the *recording parameters* (*filters, sensitivity, paper speed,* or *time base*), the *montage,* and the *calibration signal.* If you have read the first part of the book, you are already well versed with each of these terms.

Now, let's get to the exciting part: the brain waves!

Spend a few seconds staring at the first page. Observe and admire the myriad of squiggly lines that makes up the EEG. You're looking at your patient's cerebral cortex in action and there is no other test that can do this. As you look at the page, some activities will become obvious, they will catch your eye. This is what we shall refer to as the foreground. In contrast, the remainder of the page is the background. You must do this each time you see a record, until it becomes second nature. Remember, the foreground is what stares back at you when you look at the page and the rest is all background. Some beginners may find this exercise difficult at first: I did. Our mind can be easily overwhelmed by the sheer amount of activity on a page, which makes separating foreground from the background confusing.

I can assure you, that these difficulties will resolve with time and practice. One helpful exercise is to apply this concept to artwork. Go look at a few paintings. Ask yourself "Who are the main protagonists in the scene?," that's foreground, the scenery behind them is background. One of my all-time favorite paintings is in Figure 9.1, *The Fog Warning* by Winslow Homer, painted in 1884. It now resides in the Museum of Fine Arts in Boston [3].

What do you see? The fisherman, his boat, and catch are the foreground. The sea, the waves, their crests, the approaching fog, and the sky are the background. Try this yourself on some of your favorite paintings. In no time you will be a master at distinguishing the foreground from the background.

Now, let's come back to the EEG.

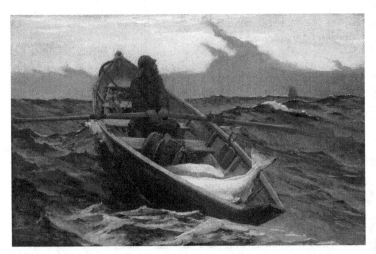

Figure 9.1 Winslow Homer, *The Fog Warning/Halibut Fishing*, 1885. Oil on canvas.

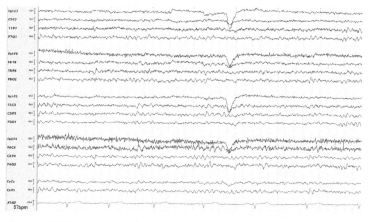

Figure 9.2 Thirty-two-year-old gentleman with an intact cranium.

In Figure 9.2 is the EEG of a 32-year-old man in normal wakefulness with an undamaged cranium. During your moment of studied reflection, mentally note the large positive (downward) deflections in the frontal channels (Fp1-F7, Fp1-F3) and (Fp2-F8, Fp2-F4), also note the short fast spiky pattern that is seen in channels Fp2-F4 and F4-C4 (Common electrode F4). These are the foreground features on this page and the remainder is background. In Figure 9.3, I have marked out the components of the foreground in this page. Currently, there is no need to worry about what these waveforms mean. All you need to be able to do, is *tell the foreground, apart from the underlying background.*

Once you have identified the foreground and the background, we will describe each of these in further detail. Conventionally, most readers will first describe the background. Arguably, it is the more important part of the record, as it tells us the state of the underlying cortex. Therefore, let's first concentrate on the background.

To *describe the background,* use six key features [4]. They are as follows:

1. symmetry
2. continuity
3. voltage
4. organization
5. reactivity or variability
6. sleep architecture

We will learn about each of these in Chapter 10.

Once we have described the background, we come to the *foreground.*

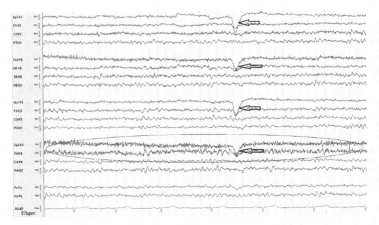

Figure 9.3 Foreground components include the large positive deflections (arrows) in the frontopolar electrodes (Fp1 and Fp2) and the short fast spiky pattern (circled) in channel F4.

Foreground components should be categorized as either cerebral activity or artifact.

1. *Activity:* Activity refers to cerebral activity. These waveforms are generated by the cerebral cortex. Cerebral activity should be described by *location* (generalized, lateralized, focal, or multifocal), *occurrence* (sporadic or repetitive), and *morphology* (slow waves or sharp/spike waves). You will learn to identify and describe each of these waveforms in Chapter 11.

2. *Artifacts:* Artifacts are contaminants. These patterns are not produced by the brain. External or nonphysiological artifacts are those that originate from outside sources, such as the ringing of a telephone. Internal or physiological artifacts originate from within the patient's body, but from sites other than the brain, such as eye blink artifact or EKG artifact. The main purpose of recognizing artifacts is to avoid confusing them with cerebral activity. Chapter 12 describes commonly encountered artifacts.

After describing the cerebral activity, assign a motive, is it normal or abnormal?

1. *Normal variants:* These are normal patterns that tend to stand out and appear abnormal. Many occur during drowsiness and sleep. Recognizing these variants avoids mistaking them for abnormalities. Chapter 13 describes normal variants.

2. *Abnormalities:* Cerebral activity that indicates an underlying abnormality should be described as mentioned, that is, by location, occurrence, and morphology, that is, slow or sharp waves.

   i. Certain abnormalities are associated with epileptic seizures/epilepsy; these are called epileptogenic abnormalities. Epileptogenic abnormalities are usually sharp in appearance (spike or sharp wave), hence they may also be called epileptiform abnormalities (or epileptic discharges). However, this isn't absolute. Certain slow rhythmic patterns, which are not epileptiform, may also be epileptogenic abnormalities. For example, temporal intermittent rhythmic delta (TIRDA) and occipital intermittent rhythmic delta activity (ORIDA) are associated with epileptic seizures. Sporadic abnormalities are described in Chapter 14, while repetitive abnormalities are described in Chapter 15.

   ii. So, what is a seizure? When an abnormal pattern transforms its speed (frequency), shape (morphology), or spreads (location) it is called *evolution.* Evolution is the electrographic hallmark of a seizure, but all evolution isn't a seizure. Note that I purposely left out amplitude; changes in amplitude alone do not constitute evolution in the context of whether a pattern could be a seizure. Evolution must be in either frequency, morphology, or location. Waveforms that represent ongoing seizure activity are called ictal patterns (Chapter 16).

Finally, we must know the *activation procedures.* These are performed to provoke epileptic activity. The two most commonly performed procedures are *photic stimulation* and *hyperventilation* as described in Chapter 17.

Just before you finish, there are a few final features to look at:

1. *EKG channel:* This is usually a single channel electrocardiogram that is useful to detect abnormalities in heart rhythm.

2. *Technologist's notes:* Always make a point to simultaneously look through the technologist's log notes as you interpret the EEG. These include information such as a change in the patient's mental state, movements, or other pertinent clinical descriptions. Looking at the *video*, if available, also allows the reader to make clinical correlations [5].

Using the above approach may seem a bit tedious at first, but with a little practice, the entire exercise will become intuitive.

You will be able to rapidly analyze the EEG.

Chapter Summary

Go through the following checklist when reading an EEG:

1. Confirm the patient's identity, age, state(s) of recording, and the presence of any skull defects.
2. Confirm the technical parameters of including the filter settings, sensitivity, paper speed, or time base. Note the montage you are reading in and the calibration signal.
3. Identify the background from the foreground.
4. Describe the background based on symmetry, continuity, voltage, organization, reactivity (or variability), and sleep architecture.
5. Categorize the foreground components as cerebral activity or artifact.
6. Describe cerebral activity based on its location (general, lateral, or focal), occurrence (sporadic or repetitive), and morphology (slow or sharp).
7. Then categorize the activity as normal (normal variant) or abnormality.
8. Decide whether the abnormality is epileptogenic (associated with seizures) or not. If epileptogenic, is it ictal (ongoing seizure). Epileptogenic abnormalities are not always epileptiform (spike or sharp waves). Evolution is the hallmark of electrographic seizure activity. Remember that isolated changes in amplitude are not evolution.
9. Look for the use of any provocation methods, such as hyperventilation and photic stimulation, and their effect on the EEG.
10. Before you finish up, make sure you've looked at the single channel EKG, technologist's log, and video (if available).

Now you can correlate your findings with your patient's clinical presentation.

References

1. Cobb WA, Guiloff RJ, Cast J. Breach rhythm: the EEG related to skull defects. *Electroencephalography and Clinical Neurophysiology.* 1979 Sep 1;47(3):251–71.

2. Otsubo H, Steinlin M, Hwang PA, et al. Positive epileptiform discharges in children with neuronal migration disorders. *Pediatric Neurology.* 1997 Jan 1;16(1):23–31.

3. Museum of Fine Arts, Boston.

4. Hirsch LJ, LaRoche SM, Gaspard N, et al. American clinical neurophysiology society's standardized critical care EEG terminology: 2012 version. *Journal of Clinical Neurophysiology.* 2013;30(1):1–27.

5. American Electroencephalographic Society Ad Hoc Guidelines Committee. Minimum technical requirements for performing clinical electroencephalography. *Journal of Clinical Neurophysiology.* 1994;11:2–5.

Background

The electrographic background reflects the patient's state and level of consciousness.

You can describe it based on the following six features:

1. symmetry
2. continuity
3. voltage
4. organization (anterior–posterior gradient, predominant frequencies, and posterior-dominant rhythm)
5. reactivity (or variability)
6. sleep architecture

Let us understand the usage of each term with its clinical significance.

Symmetry

To determine if the EEG background is symmetric over both hemispheres, *contrast their frequencies and amplitudes.*

First, use a longitudinal bipolar montage to compare the hemispheric frequencies and then use a referential montage to compare their amplitudes [1].

The background may be

1. symmetric
2. mildly asymmetric (if there is frequency asymmetry of less than 1 Hz or consistent amplitude asymmetry of less than 50%)
3. markedly asymmetric (if there is frequency asymmetry of more than 1 Hz or consistent amplitude asymmetry of more than 50%)

The normal background is symmetric, a mild physiological asymmetry with the dominant hemisphere having a slightly lower amplitude than the non-dominant side is within normal limits. Figure 10.1 shows a markedly asymmetric left hemispheric background.

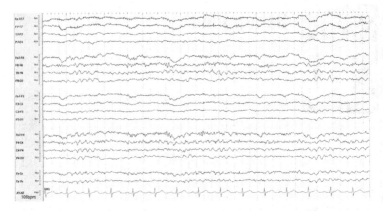

Figure 10.1 Seventy-one-year-old woman with left cerebral hemi atrophy, leptomeningeal thickening, and gyral calcifications from Sturge–Weber syndrome. There is marked asymmetry both in amplitude and frequency over the left hemisphere.

Significance

1. There is physiological asymmetry. The nondominant hemisphere (commonly right) may have a slightly higher background amplitude compared to the dominant hemisphere (commonly left). Conversely, a higher dominant background or a markedly increased nondominant background is abnormal [2].

2. Skull defects (e.g., craniotomy) leads to higher amplitudes and the presence of faster frequencies over the region, underlying activity may also appear sharper. This is called a breach effect [3]. Figure 10.2 shows a left temporal breach effect.

3. Subdural lesions (e.g., hematoma or fluid collections) predominantly dampen the amplitude of cerebral activity, they may also cause slowing.

4. Structural lesions (e.g., strokes or tumors) predominantly cause slowing of cerebral activity, they may also dampen amplitude.

5. Ictal activity may be associated with faster frequencies and higher amplitudes, while slowing and/or suppression is typical of postictal states.

6. A combination of higher amplitudes but slower frequencies may be the result of a breach effect with an underlying structural lesion (e.g., craniotomy for tumor).

If the background is markedly asymmetric, other features such as continuity, voltage, reactivity (or variability), and sleep architecture should be described separately for each hemisphere [2].

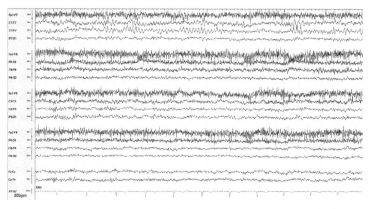

Figure 10.2 Sixty-two-year-old man with a left craniotomy for evacuation of a subdural hematoma. There is breach effect over the left temporal region (T7 channel).

Continuity

This refers to *periods of attenuation or suppression.*

Attenuation is the periodic dampening of amplitudes to less than half of the remaining background but remaining greater than 10 uV.

Suppression is severe attenuation, where amplitude of cerebral activity is less than 10 uV.

The background may be

1. continuous – without attenuation/suppression
2. nearly continuous – occasional, very brief periods of attenuation/suppression
3. discontinuous – frequent periods of attenuation/suppression that make up less than half the recording
4. burst-suppressed (or burst-attenuated), periods of attenuation/suppression for more than half of record:

   - always specify the typical duration of the bursts and the interburst intervals
   - also specify if the bursts are symmetric, synchronous and identical or nonidentical in appearance [1]

The normal background is continuous. Figures 10.3 (nearly continuous), 10.4 (discontinuous), and 10.5 (burst-suppression) show increasing levels of background discontinuity.

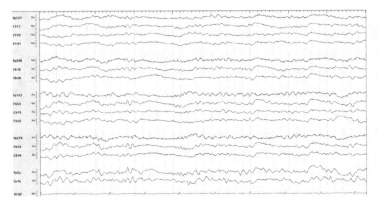

Figure 10.3 Forty-five-year-old woman sedated for episodes of agitation showing a near-continuous background. Note the brief (1 s) period of diffuse background suppression.

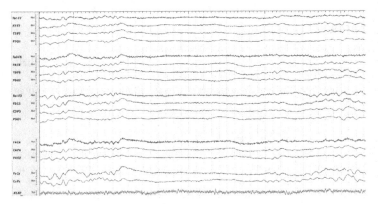

Figure 10.4 Discontinuous background with increasing sedation in the same patient as in Figure 10.3.

Significance

1. Discontinuity is an electrographic marker of the severity of encephalopathy. Longer interburst intervals (with shorter bursts) are associated with a greater depth of encephalopathy. It is nonspecific to etiology

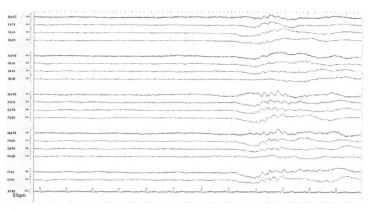

Figure 10.5 Burst-suppressed background with increased sedation in the same patient as in Figure 10.3.

but commonly associated with the use of sedative agents, metabolic disturbances (typically reversible) and in postanoxic states (typically irreversible) [4].

2. Highly epileptiform bursts (HEBs) are bursts with multiple epileptiform abnormalities (spike or sharp waves). These may be associated with ongoing underlying ictal activity such as partially suppressed or refractory status epilepticus [1,5]. Figure 10.6 shows HEBs in a patient being treated for generalized status epilepticus.

3. Burst-suppression with identical bursts is a distinct EEG pattern associated with poor outcomes in post anoxic coma. Here almost all the bursts in the record look stereotypical or identical to one another [6].

Voltage

The overall voltage or amplitude of the background cerebral activity is also called "development."

Determine the background voltage by measuring the height of the activity from peak to trough on a longitudinal bipolar montage.

Normal cerebral background voltage is variable, but greater than 20 uV (usually 30–40 uV). A low-voltage background is less than 20 uV and a suppressed background is less than 10 uV [1].

If the background is discontinuous (e.g., burst-suppressed), the background voltage refers to the amplitude of bursts [1]. Figure 10.7 shows a suppressed background.

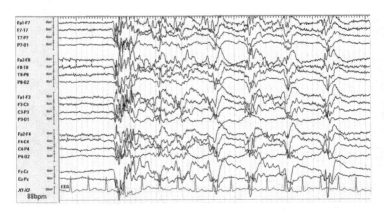

Figure 10.6 Thirty-five-year-old man being treated for generalized status epilepticus post cardiac arrest. Highly epileptiform bursts (HEBs) consisting of generalized discharges seen within bursts.

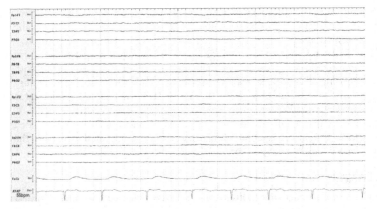

Figure 10.7 Sixty-eight-year-old woman post cardiac arrest showing a suppressed background.

Significance

1. Low background voltage is a nonspecific electrographic marker of diffuse cortical dysfunction. This may result from several different etiologies including hypoperfusion, alcoholism, medications, and metabolic

disturbances and neurodegeneration (e.g., dementia). Occasionally, it may be entirely normal.
2. The depth of suppression correlates with the severity of the encephalopathy. Complete suppression is typical with anesthetic or post anoxic coma [7].

Organization

This is the overall layout of the background cerebral activity; it may be further described based on the following three features:

1. *Anterior–posterior gradient:* Look for an anterior to posterior gradient of voltages and frequencies such that the lower amplitudes and faster frequencies are seen in the anterior channels and the higher amplitudes and slower frequencies are seen in the posterior channels. A normal, well-organized background has an appreciable anterior–posterior gradient [1].
2. *Predominant frequencies:* Specify the typical frequency of the background cerebral activity (usually alpha, theta, or delta) during maximal wakefulness, which may be after stimulation in a poorly responsive patient. Other frequencies such as beta may also be present (e.g., moderate or excess beta is present symmetrically). The predominant background frequency during normal wakefulness is alpha.
3. *Posterior-dominant rhythm (PDR):* If present, it should be described. Normally, an alpha frequency posterior-dominant rhythm is seen in the waking state that is reactive to eye closure [1,2].

A well-organized background (normal) is shown in Figure 10.8. Note the distinct anterior–posterior gradient, predominant alpha frequency, and a reactive posterior-dominant rhythm of 10 Hz. Figure 10.9 shows a poorly organized background with loss of anterior–posterior gradient, predominantly delta and theta slowing and absence of posterior-dominant rhythm.

Significance

1. Loss of an anterior–posterior gradient, predominantly slower frequencies (theta or delta), and the absence of a posterior-dominant rhythm constitute a deterioration of background organization.
2. Poorly organized background is a nonspecific electrographic marker of the severity of cerebral dysfunction. A return of background organization correlates with the resolution of cerebral dysfunction.

Reactivity (or Variability)

Reactivity refers to changes of background cerebral activity (either amplitude or frequency) in response to external stimulation. Stimulation should be specified and advanced in a graded fashion (auditory, such as name-calling,

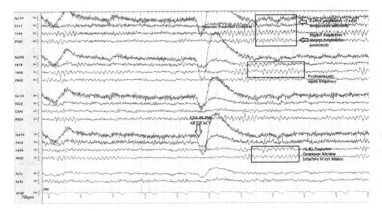

Figure 10.8 Forty-five-year-old man with episodic tinnitus showing features of a well-organized background.

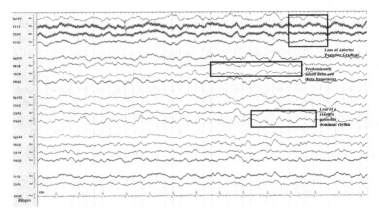

Figure 10.9 Fifty-six-year-old woman with hepatic encephalopathy showing loss of background organization.

to noxious, such as nail bed pressure). Stimulation induced foreground activities may also emerge [1]. If reactivity has not been tested, or is absent – the reader should assess the record for variability.

Variability refers to the natural transformations of background cerebral activity with fluctuations in the level of alertness or arousals. These tend to be

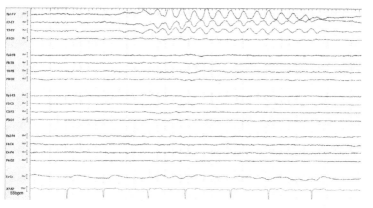

Figure 10.10 Seventy-two-year-old woman in a coma showing a rhythmic left temporal artifact upon sternal stimulation.

spontaneous (without stimulation) and sustained (at least a minute in duration). Variability is best assessed during silent periods and care should be taken to limit artifacts (e.g., respirators or IV pumps).

Normal background is reactive (e.g., eye blinks) and variable (e.g., state change). Figure 10.10 shows a sternal rub artifact over the left temporal channels, this action elicits a low-voltage burst of diffuse mixed delta and theta slowing in an otherwise suppressed background, as shown in Figure 10.11.

Significance

Reactivity (or variability) is typically associated with favorable clinical outcomes irrespective of etiology but the lack of a standardized approach to assessment and interpretation can be a limitation [7].

Sleep Architecture

The reader should assess the record for the presence of stage II sleep architecture (sleep spindles and/or K complexes). These constitute further evidence of physiological state changes. Absent or asymmetric stage II sleep architecture is usually abnormal. Figure 10.12 shows symmetric sleep spindles in a sedated patient.

Significance

1. The presence of normal sleep architecture is typically regarded as a favorable prognostic marker, irrespective of etiology [8].
2. Asymmetric K complexes or spindles may be seen with cerebral dysfunction or damage [9].

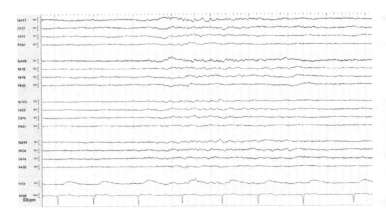

Figure 10.11 Sternal stimulation is shortly followed by a brief burst of low-amplitude activity in the same patient (Figure 10.10) indicating reactivity.

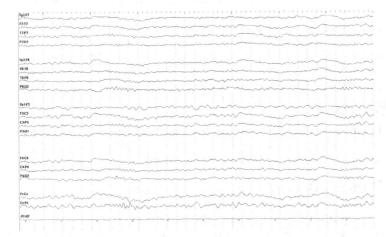

Figure 10.12 Fifty-eight-year-old woman in a propofol-induced coma showing symmetric spindles.

3. Spindle coma refers to a nonspecific electrographic pattern characterized by an abundance of spindle activity and other sleep transients in comatose individuals [8].
4. Anesthetic agents such as propofol may induce spindle activity [10].

Chapter Summary

You can describe the electrographic background described based on the following features:

1. *Symmetry:* It may be symmetric, mildly asymmetric, or markedly asymmetric. Mild asymmetry of the dominant hemisphere may be physiologic.
2. *Continuity:* It may be continuous, nearly continuous, discontinuous, or burst-suppressed. Attenuation is the periodic dampening of amplitudes by less than half the remaining background while suppression is when the amplitude falls below 10 uV.
3. *Voltage:* It may be normal (above 20 uV), low voltage (20–10 uV), or suppressed (less than 10 uV).
4. *Organization:* A well-organized background has an anterior–posterior gradient, predominantly alpha frequencies, and a reactive posterior-dominant rhythm (PDR). The loss of either or all these features results in a deterioration in background organization.
5. *Reactivity (or variability):* Reactivity refers to changes in background amplitude or frequency in response to external stimulation, while variability refers to spontaneous fluctuations in the patient's level of alertness. Always specify the stimulation used to test reactivity and advance it in a graded manner. Reactivity (or variability) of the background are associated with favorable clinical outcomes.
6. *Presence of stage II sleep architecture such as spindles and K complexes should be noted:* They may be symmetric or asymmetric. Sleep spindles may be induced by anesthetics such as propofol. Sleep spindles and K complexes are associated with favorable clinical outcomes.

References

1. Hirsch LJ, LaRoche SM, Gaspard N, et al. American clinical neurophysiology society's standardized critical care EEG terminology: 2012 version. *Journal of Clinical Neurophysiology.* 2013 Feb 1;**30**(1):1–27.

2. Britton JW, Frey LC, Hopp JL, et al. *Electroencephalography (EEG): an introductory text and atlas of normal and abnormal findings in adults, children, and infants.* American Epilepsy Society, Chicago; 2016.

3. Cobb WA, Guiloff RJ, Cast J. Breach rhythm: the EEG related to skull defects. *Electroencephalography and Clinical Neurophysiology.* 1979 Sep 1;**47**(3):251–71.

4. Tsetsou S, Oddo M, Rossetti AO. Clinical outcome after a reactive hypothermic EEG following cardiac arrest. *Neurocritical Care.* 2013 Dec 1;**19**(3):283–6.

5. Thompson SA, Hantus S. Highly epileptiform bursts are associated with seizure recurrence. *Journal of Clinical Neurophysiology.* 2016 Feb 1;**33**(1):66–71.

6. Hofmeijer J, Tjepkema-Cloostermans MC, van Putten MJ. Burst-suppression with identical bursts: a distinct EEG pattern with poor outcome in postanoxic coma. *Clinical Neurophysiology.* 2014 May 1;**125**(5):947–54.

7. Hofmeijer J, van Putten MJ. EEG in postanoxic coma: prognostic and diagnostic value. *Clinical Neurophysiology.* 2016 Apr 1;**127**(4):2047–55.

8. Azabou E, Navarro V, Kubis N, et al. Value and mechanisms of EEG reactivity in the prognosis of patients with impaired consciousness: a systematic review. *Critical Care.* 2018 Dec 1;**22**(1):184.

9. Clemens B, Ménes A. Sleep spindle asymmetry in epileptic patients. *Clinical Neurophysiology.* 2000 Dec 1;**111**(12):2155–9.

10. Huotari AM, Koskinen M, Suominen K, et al. Evoked EEG patterns during burst suppression with propofol. *British Journal of Anaesthesia.* 2004 Jan 1;**92**(1):18–24.

Foreground (How to Describe an Abnormality)

Waveforms in the foreground may be artifact or cerebral activity (normal variants or abnormalities).

Each type of waveform observed may be identified and classified based on three key features:

1. *Location:* Is the waveform predominantly diffuse (generalized), hemispheric (lateralized), focal (regional), or multifocal?
2. *Occurrence:* Is the waveform sporadic (single or abundant but occurs randomly) or repetitive (recurs in rhythmic or periodic pattern)?
3. *Morphology:* Is it pointed (spike or sharp) or blunt (slow wave) in appearance?

For example, the term generalized periodic discharge (GPD) denotes a sharp or spike wave (discharge) that is generalized in location and occurs repetitively in a periodic fashion as shown in Figure 11.1.

These key terms are simply introduced here, they are explained in the following chapters.

After you have described a waveform based on the above three key features of location, occurrence, and morphology, use the following additional modifiers to qualify your description [1]:

1. prevalence
2. duration
3. amplitude
4. frequency

The appropriate usage of each of these terms is explained below. They are particularly useful in describing abnormalities seen on continuous EEG monitoring in the critically ill patients [1]. It is important to note that these modifiers are used in context of the entire record or epoch and not an individual page of the EEG.

Prevalence

This denotes the approximate amount (percentage) of the specific waveform in the record:

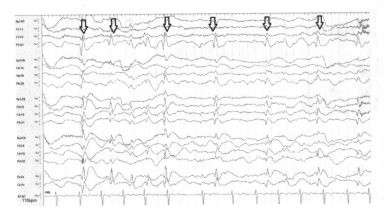

Figure 11.1 Sixty-two-year-old man in a coma showing occipital-predominant generalized periodic discharges (GPDs).

1. continuous, if the waveform occurs contiguously through almost the entire record.
2. intermittent, if the waveform occurs in parts during the record. Intermittent waveforms may be further described as abundant (>50%), frequent (49%–10%), occasional (9%–1%), or rare (<1%), depending on approximately how often they are observed during the entire record [1].

Figure 11.1 shows "continuous" generalized periodic discharges, while Figure 11.2 shows "intermittent" discharges.

Duration

This is the typical length of time for which - intermittent patterns observed in the record, this is particularly useful in continuous EEG monitoring. Intermittent patterns may be further described as very long (hours), long (minutes), or brief (seconds), depending on their approximate duration [1].

For example, Figure 11.2 shows a very brief (1 s) burst of frontally predominant generalized spike wave discharges.

Amplitude

Measure the amplitude (absolute amplitude) from the peak to the trough of the waveform (positive to negative peak) and not peak to baseline. It is best to measure the amplitude in longitudinal bipolar montage (in the channel it is best seen). Figure 11.3 shows the correct method to measure the amplitude of a waveform.

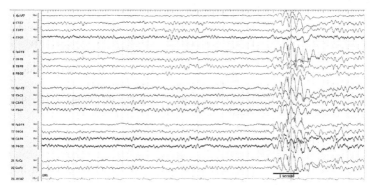

Figure 11.2 Thirty-four-year-old man with epilepsy showing intermittent very brief (1 s) frontally predominant generalized spike wave discharges (GSW).

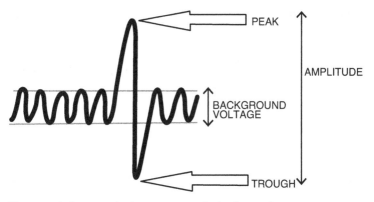

Figure 11.3 Correct method to measure amplitude of a waveform.

The typical amplitude can then be described as low (less than 20 uV), medium (less than 50 uV), or high (more than 200 uV) [1].

Frequency

The rate (typical and range) should be specified for a pattern to the nearest 0.5/s division [1]. For example, in Figure 11.2, the discharges typically occur at a frequency of 4 Hz (four times per second).

Reporting the Foreground Abnormality

When reporting the waveform, the modifiers (prevalence, duration, amplitude, and frequency) should precede the three key features of location, occurrence, and morphology.

For example, Figure 11.1 shows "continuous, long duration, high-amplitude, 2–1 Hz, occipitally predominant generalized periodic discharges" and Figure 11.2 shows "intermittent, very brief, high-amplitude, 4 Hz, frontally predominant generalized spike wave discharges."

Chapter Summary

1. First identify the foreground abnormality (or activity) based on three key features of location (generalized, lateralized, focal, or multifocal), occurrence (sporadic or repetitive), and morphology (sharp or blunt).
2. Next, qualify your description with the modifiers of prevalence, duration, amplitude, and frequency.
3. When reporting the waveform, the modifiers (prevalence, duration, amplitude, and frequency) should precede the three key features of location, occurrence, and morphology.

Reference

1. Hirsch LJ, LaRoche SM, Gaspard N, et al. American clinical neurophysiology society's standardized critical care EEG terminology: 2012 version. *Journal of Clinical Neurophysiology*. 2013 Feb 1;**30**(1):1–27.

Chapter 12

Common Artifacts

Artifacts are noncerebral waveforms that mimic cerebral activity. Excess artifact may hide underlying abnormalities.

When artifacts originate from within the body (organs other than the brain) they are called internal or physiologic artifacts. Those originating outside the body are called external or nonphysiologic artifacts [1].

Closely examine the bedside environment either in person or on video to identify the cause. Numerous external and internal artifacts can occur, some commonly encountered ones are described below.

Common External Artifacts

Electrode Artifact

High electrode impedance or a sudden change in impedance (electrode pop) leads to artifact in the affected channels. Often nearby alternating current sources such as electrical devices (e.g., dialysis machines, pumps, beds) will also reflect in these problem electrodes causing more artifact (60 Hz artifact).

They have a variable appearance but regardless of montage electrode artifacts are limited to the channels containing the problem electrode (no field) [2].

Significance

1. They may be spiky, periodic, or rhythmic and may mimic epileptogenic or ictal patterns.
2. Electrode artifact (e.g., 60 Hz) can cause unusual patterns in several channels, these can sometimes mimic cerebral background activity. Turning off the 60 Hz filter reveals the underlying artifact.
3. Fix or replace the electrode, turn off any nearby devices (such as pumps), or use a filter to decrease this artifact.

Figure 12.1 shows spiky appearing electrode artifact at T8 and Figure 12.2 shows "pop" artifact at P7.

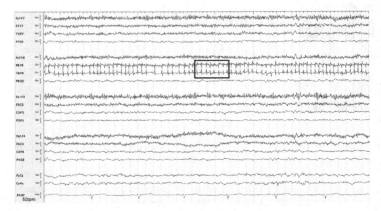

Figure 12.1 Thirty-eight-year-old man with alcohol intoxication, spiky periodic T8 electrode artifact.

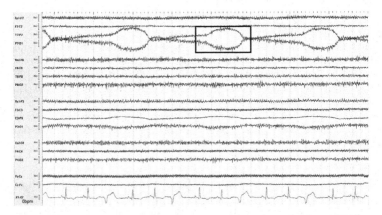

Figure 12.2 Seventy-two-year-old man in a coma, "electrode pop" artifact at P7. Note the irregular heart rate.

Sweat Artifact

This occurs due to a moist scalp. It is typically a slow sinusoidal delta pattern that can appear in a single or multiple channel [3].

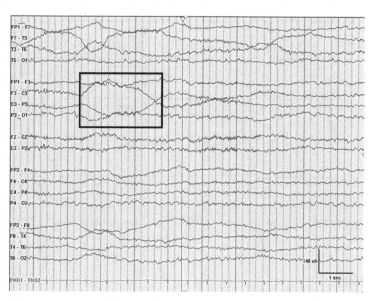

Figure 12.3 Fifty-seven-year-old man with encephalopathy, sweat artifact in multiple channels.

Significance

1. May mimic slow lateral eye movements (esp. in F7 and F8) or generalized rhythmic delta activity (GRDA).
2. Wipe the scalp, cool the patient, or use a low-frequency filter to decrease this artifact.

Figure 12.3 shows sweat artifact in multiple channels.

Ventilator Artifact

This typically leads to a regular paced slower waveform (single or burst-like). Occasionally, faster activity may result from fluid in the tubing. Commonly affects the anterior channels but variable in location and appearance. Figure 12.4 shows a periodic appearing ventilator artifact occurring every 6 s and corresponding to the set respiratory rate [3].

Significance

1. Monitoring the ventilation rate either using a separate channel (mouth electrodes) or at bedside helps identify the artifact.
2. May mimic bursts of cerebral activity in comatose patients.

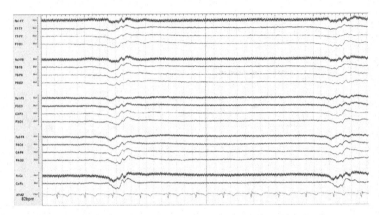

Figure 12.4 Eighty-year-old woman in a coma, slow-paced ventilator artifact.

Others

Rhythmic artifact may result from telephone ringing, bed-percussion, or devices such as Continuous Renal Replacement Therapy (CRRT), and Extracorporeal Membrane Oxygenation (ECMO).

Cardiopulmonary resuscitation, sternal rub, chest percussion, tooth brushing, and other maneuvers also result in fast rhythmic artifacts that may mimic ictal activity [3]. Figure 12.5 shows diffuse (including EKG channel) rhythmic appearing artifact from brushing teeth.

Common Internal Artifacts

The eyes, tongue, heart, and muscles are common causes of internal artifact.

Eye Artifacts

Vertical Eye Movements (Includes Eye Blinks): The eye is a dipole with the cornea charged positive and the retina charged negative. With lid closure the cornea rolls up toward the frontopolar channels (Fp1 and Fp2) due to Bell's phenomena, leading to a large downward deflection (positive is down) in those channels. Eye opening will have the opposite effect (upward deflection). Figure 12.6 shows eye blink artifact and Figure 12.7 shows vertical eye movement artifact in the Fp1 and Fp2 channels.

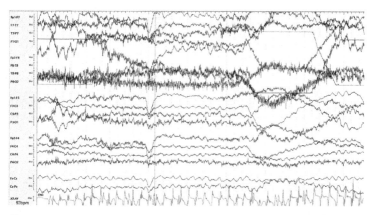

Figure 12.5 Thirty-five-year-old man with shaking spells, diffuse rhythmic toothbrushing artifact.

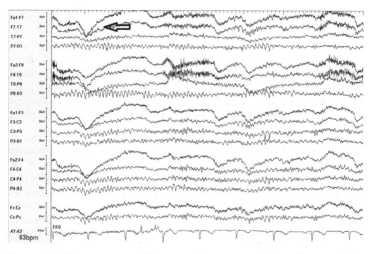

Figure 12.6 Thirty-seven-year-old woman with seizures, eye blink artifact in the frontopolar (Fp) channels.

Significance

1. Vertical nystagmus or ocular bobbing may also result in a similar artifact. Vertical nystagmus has a sharp upward defection (corresponds to

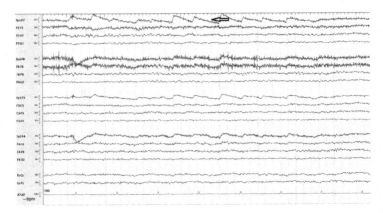

Figure 12.7 Thirty-five-year-old man with shaking spells, vertical eye movement artifact in the frontopolar (Fp) channels.

a quick down phase) and slow downward deflection (slower return to up gaze).
2. Eye lid flutter may mimic frontally predominant generalized rhythmic delta activity (GRDA). However, unlike GRDA, ocular artifacts don't extend beyond the frontopolar derivations. Figure 12.8 shows prominent eye flutter artifact.
3. In rare circumstances inferior orbital electrodes may be used to confirm vertical eye movement artifact where the waveforms are always out of phase compared to the frontopolar channels [1,2].

Lateral Eye Movements: Similar principles apply (the cornea is positive relative to the retina), but these waveforms are seen in F7 and F8. If the eyes look to the left (F7) then the positive cornea causes a downward deflection in the F7 channel and a corresponding upward deflection in F8. When looking to the right (F8) there is an upward deflection in F7 and a downward deflection in F8. Figure 12.9 shows lateral eye movement artifact during wakefulness. Lateral rectus spikes characterized by a small artifactual spike (commonly in the F7/F8 channel) may precede lateral eye movements [1,2].

Significance

1. Lateral nystagmus (e.g., due to seizures) may cause similar artifact. Figure 12.10 shows artifact produced by lateral nystagmus in the left eye (F7 channel).

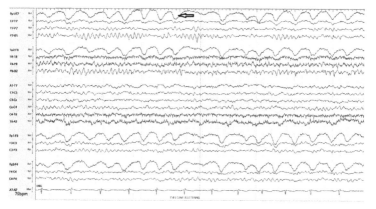

Figure 12.8 Twenty-eight-year-old woman with anxious spells, eye flutter artifact in the frontopolar (Fp) channels.

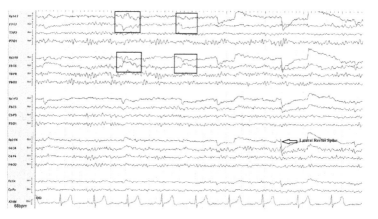

Figure 12.9 Thirty-five-year-old man with shaking spells, horizontal eye movement artifact in F7/F8 and lateral rectus spikes.

2. Rapid eye movement (REM) sleep results in lateral eye movement artifact but without eye blinks. Figure 12.11 shows lateral eye movements during REM sleep.

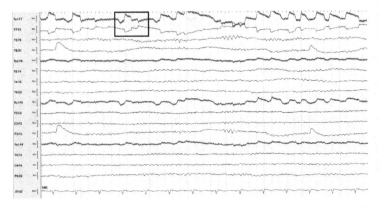

Figure 12.10 Sixty-four-year-old man with cardiac arrest, left eye lateral nystagmus (F7) artifact.

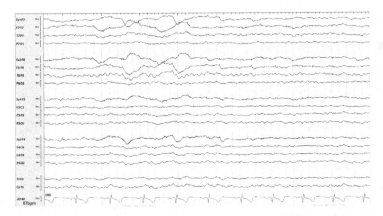

Figure 12.11 Forty-five-year-old man in rapid eye movement (REM) sleep, horizontal eye movement artifact in F7/F8.

3. Slow lateral eye movements (rowing eyes) result in out-of-phase slow sinusoidal patterns in F7 and F8 and are a normal feature of drowsiness. Figure 12.12 shows slow lateral eye movement artifact during drowsiness.

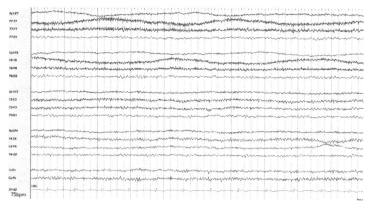

Figure 12.12 Forty-seven-year-old woman in drowsiness, slow rowing eye movement artifact at F7/F8.

Tongue (Glossopharyngeal) Artifact

The tongue is a large muscle with its tip relatively negative compared to its base. Tongue movements (such as eating, swallowing, or hyperventilation). This appears as a burst of frontally predominant high-amplitude delta slowing. Typically, there is some superimposed muscle artifact seen. It is best appreciated in the frontopolar channels but unlike ocular artifacts has a wide field that may extend to the posterior channels [2]. Figure 12.13 shows glossopharyngeal artifact while talking.

Significance

1. It may be confused with frontally predominant generalized rhythmic delta activity (GRDA).
2. The artifact may be reproduced by repeating lingual sounds such as "la-la-la" or confirmed with placement of submental electrodes.
3. Sipping from a straw may also produce a similar rhythmic artifact of delta frequency that mimics GRDA. Figure 12.14 shows a generalized rhythmic artifact produced while using a drinking straw.

Cardiac Artifact

Electrocardiogram (EKG Artifact): Regular cardiac contractions can result in a periodic artifact that corresponds with the QRS complex on the electrocardiogram channel. It is most prominent in the ear referential montages.

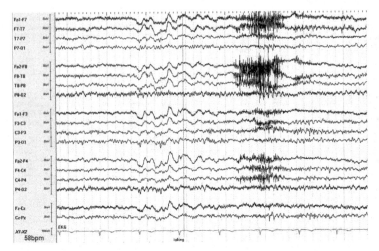

Figure 12.13 Twenty-eight-year-old woman with anxious spells, diffuse rhythmic glossopharyngeal artifact while talking.

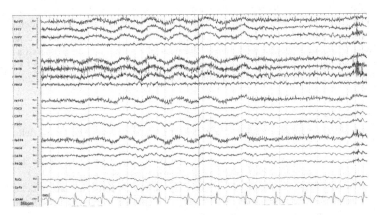

Figure 12.14 Twenty-eight-year-old woman with anxious spells, diffuse low-amplitude rhythmic artifact with sipping through a straw.

Figure 12.15 shows diffuse periodic EKG artifact that is best appreciated in the posterior channels and corresponds to the QRS complex on the EKG channel [4].

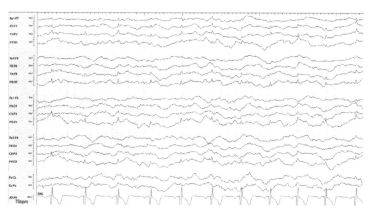

Figure 12.15 Fifty-seven-year-old man with encephalopathy, generalized periodic EKG artifact corresponding to the QRS complex on EKG channel.

Significance

1. This may be confused with periodic discharges, it is identified using the EKG channel.
2. Pacemaker may result in periodic artifacts that just precede the QRS complex.
3. Pulse artifact occurs if an electrode is placed over a pulsating vessel, it is a rhythmic or periodic artifact that follows the QRS.

Cardioballistogram artifact: This is a less commonly seen artifact that results from the rocking motion of the head and neck with forceful heart beats, it mimics slow generalized rhythmic delta activity (GRDA) but also corresponds with the QRS complex. Its duration is usually the same as the inter-QRS interval [3].

Myogenic artifact

Facial Muscles: Typically, myogenic (muscle) artifact is high amplitude, fast (>30 Hz), and spiky. It is most common in the frontal (frontalis), temporal (temporalis), and occipital (occipitalis) regions with the midline channels (Fz, Cz, and Pz) typically free from it, allowing the reader to best observe the underlying cerebral activity in these channels. It is reduced with relaxation, reassurance, and sedation. Neuromuscular blockade in intubated patients also decreases this artifact. Figure 12.16 shows right temporalis muscle artifact [1,2].

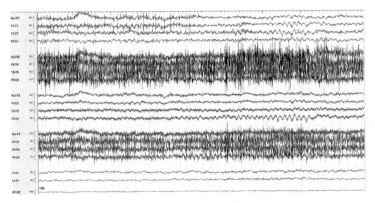

Figure 12.16 Thirty-eight-year-old man with alcohol intoxication, right temporalis muscle artifact.

Significance: Using a high-sensitivity or a high-frequency filter (70 Hz) may cause myogenic artifact to mimic beta activity. True beta, unlike muscle artifact is always seen in the central channels.

Chewing: Chewing results in a prominent generalized periodic burst of myogenic artifact that spares the midline channels. Figure 12.17 shows chewing artifact.
Significance: may resemble a generalized tonic clonic seizure [5].

Myoclonus: Cerebral myoclonus (such as postanoxic) appears as a generalized burst of spike or polyspikes (best seen in central channels) associated with diffuse myogenic artifact [6]. It may be stimulus induced. Figure 12.18 shows myoclonic artifact.

Tremors: Head tremor results in a rhythmic appearing artifact best seen in the posterior channels, while palatal tremor causes a diffuse spike wave–like artifact that is best seen with nasopharyngeal electrodes. These can be confused with electrographic seizures. Figure 12.19 shows head tremor artifact [7].

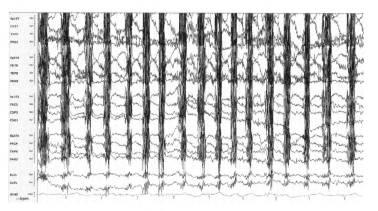

Figure 12.17 Thirty-five-year-old man with shaking spells, diffuse chewing artifact.

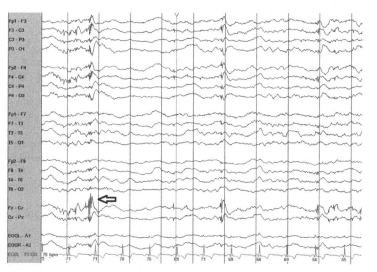

Figure 12.18 Sixty-seven-year-old man with cerebral myoclonus, myoclonic discharges best appreciated in the central channels.

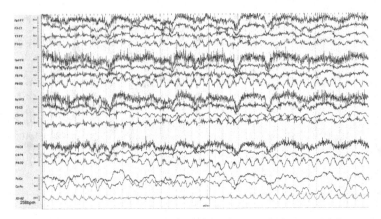

Figure 12.19 Seventy-two-year-old man with head tremor, rhythmic occipital-predominant tremor artifact.

Chapter Summary

1. Artifacts are noncerebral waveforms that may mimic or obscure cerebral activity.
2. External or nonphysiologic artifacts are produced outside the body, while internal or physiologic artifacts are produced by organs other than the brain.
3. Electrode artifacts may have a spiky, periodic, or rhythmic appearance. Characteristically, it is limited to the involved electrode with no field.
4. Sweat artifact may involve multiple channels and may be confused with lateral eye movements or GRDA.
5. Eye movement and glossopharyngeal artifact may mimic frontally predominant GRDA.
6. EKG artifact may be confused with periodic discharges. Characteristically, it corresponds to the QRS complexes.
7. Ventilatory artifact may be confused with bursts of cerebral activity. Characteristically, it corresponds to the respiratory rate.
8. Head tremor presents as occipital-predominant rhythmic artifact.
9. Maneuvers and devices such as bed-percussion, CRRT, ECMO, CPR, and even brushing teeth may lead to ictal appearing rhythmic artifacts.
10. Discharges associated with cortical myoclonus are best appreciated in the central channels, as these are relatively free of muscle artifact.

11. Chewing artifact may electrographically mimic a generalized tonic clonic seizure.
12. Close observation of the patient and the surrounding equipment either in person or on video is the key to diagnosing the cause of the artifact.

References

1. Britton JW, Frey LC, Hopp JL, et al. *Electroencephalography (EEG): an introductory text and atlas of normal and abnormal findings in adults, children, and infants.* American Epilepsy Society, Chicago; 2016.

2. Tatum WO, Dworetzky BA, Schomer DL. Artifact and recording concepts in EEG. *Journal of Clinical Neurophysiology.* 2011 Jun 1;**28**(3):252–63.

3. White DM, Van Cott CA. EEG artifacts in the intensive care unit setting. *American Journal of Electroneurodiagnostic Technology.* 2010 Mar 1;**50**(1):8–25.

4. Nakamura M, Shibasaki H. Elimination of EKG artifacts from EEG records: a new method of non-cephalic referential EEG recording. *Electroencephalography and Clinical Neurophysiology.* 1987 Jan 1;**66**(1):89–92.

5. Ebersole JS, Bridgers SL, Silva CG. Differentiation of epileptiform abnormalities from normal transients and artifacts on ambulatory cassette EEG. *American Journal of EEG Technology.* 1983 Jun 1;**23**(2):113–25.

6. Shibasaki H, Kuroiwa Y. Electroencephalographic correlates of myoclonus. *Electroencephalography and Clinical Neurophysiology.* 1975 Nov 1;**39**(5):455–63.

7. Schmitt S. Artifacts resembling seizures. In *Continuous EEG monitoring* (pp. 153–71). Springer, Cham; 2017.

Chapter 13

Normal Variants

Certain normal patterns of cerebral activity stand out from the background and resemble abnormalities. They are called "normal variants" as they have no specific clinical significance. Recognizing normal variants avoids mistaking them for epileptogenic abnormalities. Their correct identification prevents a misdiagnosis of seizures or epilepsy [1].

Normal variants can be classified based on one of three features:

1. sharp waveforms, which should be distinguished from epileptiform abnormalities
2. rhythmic waveforms, which should be distinguished from electrographic seizures
3. posterior waveforms, which should be distinguished from posterior abnormalities

Each variant can be identified based on a typical appearance, location, state, and age group as described below.

Sharp Variants

1. wickets
2. small sharp spikes (SSS)
3. positive bursts of 14 and 6 Hz
4. phantom spikes

Rhythmic Variants

1. frontal arousal rhythms (FAR)
2. rhythmic midtemporal theta of drowsiness (RMTD)
3. subclinical rhythmic electrographic (theta) discharges of adults (SREDA)
4. midline theta
5. mu rhythm
6. texting rhythm

Posterior Variants

1. lambda waves
2. posterior slow waves of youth (PSWY)
3. positive occipital sharp transients of sleep (POSTS)

Sharp Variants

These variants have a pointy (sharp) morphology. The first step is to distinguish this pattern from an epileptic discharge.

Both normal variants and epileptic discharges stand out from the background (appear taller than the adjacent waves). Being cerebral activity, both are often negative (deflect upward) and have a physiologic field [2].

Three key features that differentiate a sharp variant from an interictal epileptic discharge are as follows:

1. Normal variants, unlike epileptic discharges, don't disrupt the background, they may simply appear taller that the adjacent waves.
2. Normal variants, unlike epileptic discharges, have symmetric slopes and don't drop below the baseline.
3. Normal variants, unlike epileptic discharges, are not followed by a slow wave.

Figure 13.1 shows the differences between a sharp variant and an epileptic discharge.

Epileptic Discharge

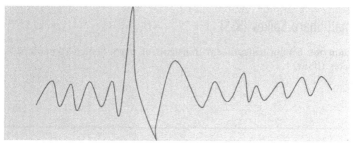

Sharp Variant

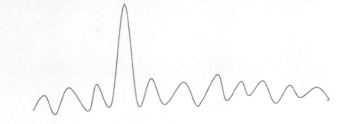

Figure 13.1 Sharp waves (epileptic discharge vs. sharp variant).

The next step is to identify the individual variant. This is done based on its appearance, location, state, and age group along with other characteristics.

Wicket Waves

Appearance: These occur in clusters (trains) with a characteristic arch shape. Single sharps also occur, but their morphology matches those in the cluster. Their amplitudes range from 60–200 uV with typical frequencies of 6–11 Hz that may resemble a Mu rhythm (described below).

Location: anterior to midtemporal, typically bilateral, and independent with shifting predominance.

State: drowsiness and light sleep

Age Group: adults

Clinical Caveat: Wicket waves are commonly misinterpreted as epileptiform abnormalities; this leads to an erroneous diagnosis of epilepsy [3]. Figure 13.2 shows a cluster of wicket waves, Figure 13.3 shows single wicket waves over the left temporal region in the same patient.

Small Sharp Spikes (SSS)

Synonyms: benign epileptiform transients of sleep, benign sporadic sleep spikes (BSSS)

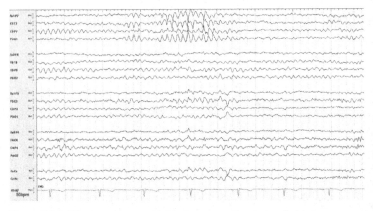

Figure 13.2 Fifty-year-old man with headache; note the cluster of wicket waves over the left temporal region.

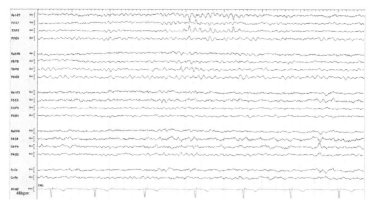

Figure 13.3 Single wicket waves over the left temporal region in the same patient.

Appearance: These occur in singles (never in trains) with a characteristic low amplitude (<50 uV) and short duration (<50 ms) with near symmetric slopes, they may be mono or diphasic and followed by a small dip in the background. They are not associated with prominent aftercoming slow waves or independent ipsilateral slowing.

Location: temporal (usually bilateral)

State: drowsiness and light sleep (disappear with deep sleep)

Age Group: adults

Best Montage: They have broad fields, best appreciated in montages with long interelectrode distances such as a contralateral ear reference [4]. Figure 13.4 shows small sharp spikes in longitudinal bipolar montage, Figure 13.5 shows the same waveforms in ear reference.

Positive Bursts of 14 Hz and 6 Hz

Synonyms: 14 and 6 Hz positive spikes, ctenoids

Appearance: Brief bursts (0.5–1 s) of alternating positive (downward) spikes and negative (upward) smooth, rounded, comb-like waveforms that resemble a sleep spindle. They may occur at 14 Hz independently, or in association with 6 Hz.

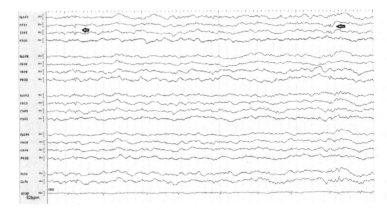

Figure 13.4 Sixty-two-year-old man with mild cognitive symptoms, small sharp spikes (SSS) during light sleep.

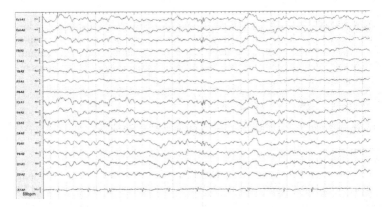

Figure 13.5 Same waveforms as in Figure 13.4 seen in ear reference.

Location: posterior temporal (shifting predominance)

State: drowsiness

Age Group: adolescents (6 to 14 years)

Best Montage: They have broad fields, best appreciated in montages with long interelectrode distances such as a contralateral ear reference [4]. Figure 13.6

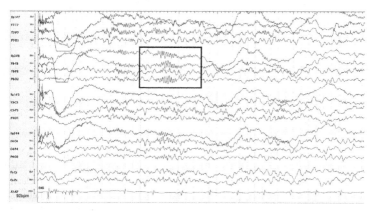

Figure 13.6 Eighteen-year-old man with starring spells, 14 Hz positive bursts with a characteristic spindle-like appearance during wakefulness.

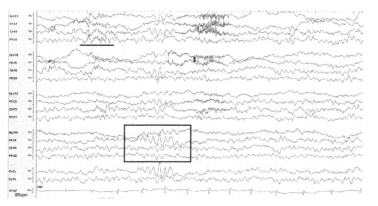

Figure 13.7 14 Hz positive bursts in association with 6 Hz waves in the same patient.

shows 14 Hz positive spikes; Figure 13.7 shows 14 Hz positive spikes in association with 6 Hz waveforms.

Phantom Spike and Wave

Synonyms: 6 Hz spike and wave discharges

Appearance: Brief (1–2 s) synchronous bursts of 5–7 Hz of tiny spikes (called phantoms as they are difficult to see) with higher amplitude slow waves.

Location: generalized, often with an anterior or posterior predominance

State: drowsiness (disappear with deep sleep)

Age Group: adolescents and adults

Best Montage: They have broad fields, so best appreciated in montages with long interelectrode distances such as a contralateral ear reference.

Clinical Caveat: There are two subtypes known by their acronyms. WHAMS (wakefulness, high amplitude, anterior, male) and FOLD (female, occipital, low amplitude, drowsy). The clinical relevance of this differentiation is unclear, however certain features such as higher amplitudes, slower frequencies (<6 Hz), occurrence during wakefulness and persistence in deep sleep suggest a higher association with seizures [4]. Figure 13.8 shows phantom spike and wave in the longitudinal bipolar montage, Figure 13.9 shows the same pattern in ear reference.

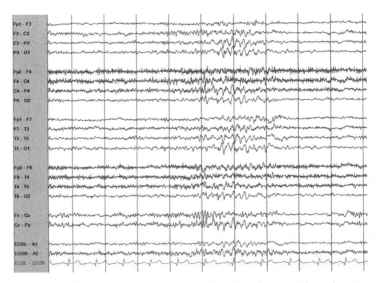

Figure 13.8 Twenty-three-year-old woman with anxiety, phantom spike, and waves most prominent over the occipital channels.

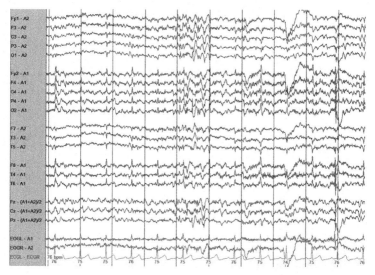

Figure 13.9 Same waveforms as seen in Figure 13.8 in ear reference.

Rhythmic Variants

These patterns consist of intermittent bursts of rhythmic activity; hence they can be mistaken for an electrographic seizure.

Three key features differentiate a "rhythmic variant" from an electrographic seizure. These are as follows:

1. Rhythmic variants have frequencies of 6 Hz or greater which do not evolve (i.e., change with time or in spatial distribution). Epileptic activity including electrographic seizures commonly speed up (crescendo) and less commonly slow down (decrescendo).
2. They disappear in deeper stages of sleep, unlike interictal epileptic seizures which are accentuated during deep sleep.
3. They are always asymptomatic.

Frontal Arousal Rhythm (FAR)

Appearance: High-amplitude rhythmic activity of 3–7 Hz occurring with arousal from sleep. May last for as long as 20 s and appear notched due

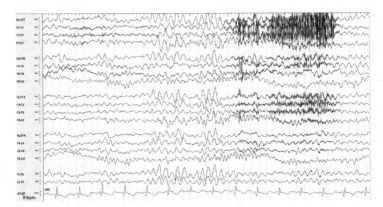

Figure 13.10 Twelve-year-old boy with headache, frontal arousal rhythm (FAR) followed by burst of muscle artifact.

to superimposed harmonics. There is a gradual increase or decrease in amplitude [4].

Location: frontal

State: arousal from sleep, disappears with wakefulness

Age Group: children
Figure 13.10 shows prominent frontal arousal rhythm, followed by muscle artifact indicative of arousal/movement.

Rhythmic Midtemporal Theta of Drowsiness (RMTD)

Synonyms: rhythmic temporal theta bursts of drowsiness, rhythmic midtemporal discharges, psychomotor variant

Appearance: Monomorphic bursts or runs of 5 to 7 Hz theta that appear sharp, flat topped or notched activity that does not show spatial or temporal evolution [4].

Location: temporal (unilateral, bilateral, or shifting)

State: drowsiness

Age Group: adolescents and adults
Figure 13.11 shows a brief left temporal RMTD; Figure 13.12 shows bitemporal RMTD with longer duration over the right temporal region.

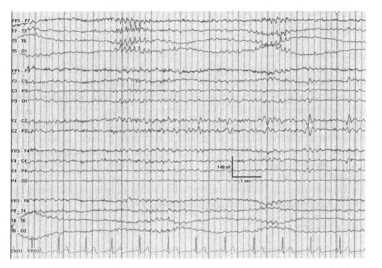

Figure 13.11 Forty-year-old woman being evaluated for seizures, burst of left temporal rhythmic midtemporal theta of drowsiness (RMTD) with a notched appearance.

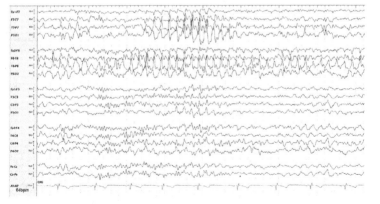

Figure 13.12 Eight-year-old boy being evaluated for seizures, bitemporal RMTD with a sharp appearance, prolonged over the right temporal region.

Subclinical Rhythmic Electrographic (Theta) Discharges of Adults (SREDA)

Appearance: Paroxysmal bursts or runs of rhythmic sharply contoured 5–7 Hz theta that is usually bilateral with a widespread distribution. Focal and unilateral forms also occur. Average duration is a little over a minute. Usually, the onset is abrupt with the page suddenly filled with repetitive monophasic sharp waveforms (Figure 13.13). It may begin with recurring semiperiodic sharp waves (Figure 13.14), at progressively shorter intervals that merge into a rhythmic pattern, usually focal over the central region (Figure 13.15). The offset, as in the onset may be abrupt (Figure 13.16) [4].

Location: Widespread with maximal amplitude over the parietal and posterior temporal region; focal and unilateral forms also occur.

State: drowsiness

Age Group: adults (typically over 50)

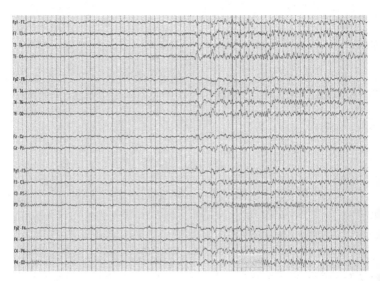

Figure 13.13 Sixty-two-year-old woman being evaluated for seizures, onset (abrupt) of diffuse sharp waveforms, characteristic of subclinical rhythmic electrographic (theta) discharges of adults (SREDA).

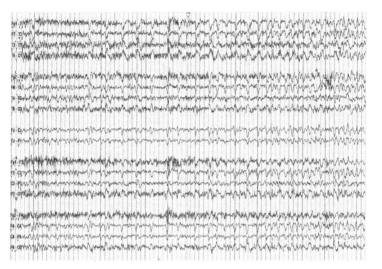

Figure 13.14 Diffuse semiperiodic sharp waves of SREDA in the same patient.

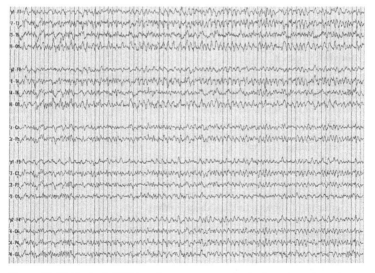

Figure 13.15 Rhythmic SREDA as the pattern progresses in the same patient.

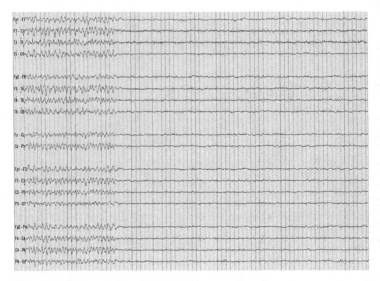

Figure 13.16 Abrupt offset of SREDA in the same patient.

Midline Theta

Synonyms: Ciganek

Appearance: Trains of focal central (vertex) rhythmic theta activity (5–7 Hz) with usually a smooth or sinusoidal appearance but can sometimes be sharply contoured or arciform. Its duration is variable, but typically waxes and wanes [4].

Location: midline (central)

State: wakefulness and drowsiness

Age Group: adults

Figure 13.17 shows a midline theta rhythm.

Mu Rhythm

Appearance: Often asymmetric and asynchronous rhythmic central alpha activity (8–10 Hz) with an arciform morphology.

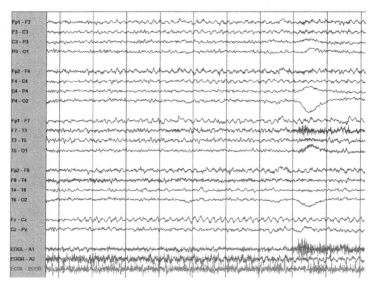

Figure 13.17 Forty-nine-year-old man with episodic movements, central midline theta (Ciganek) rhythm most prominent over the central channels (Cz).

Location: midline (central)

State: wakefulness

Age Group: adolescents and adults

Clinical Caveat: This is the resting rhythm of the sensorimotor cortex, that unlike alpha does not block with eye opening but will block with movement of the opposite extremities [4]. Figure 13.18 shows a Mu rhythm at C3 in longitudinal bipolar montage, Figure 13.19 shows the same waveform in referential montage.

Texting Rhythm

This is a recently described variant characterized by bursts of generalized rhythmic 5–6 Hz monomorphic theta activity predominantly over the frontocentral region and specifically evoked by active phone texting or smart phone use. This may represent activation of cognitive-visual-motor networks during cortical processing [5]. Figure 13.20 shows an example of "texting" rhythm.

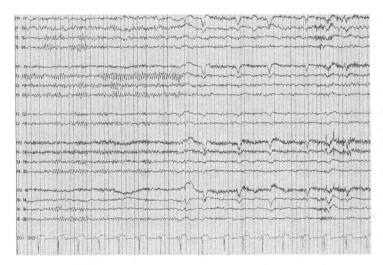

Figure 13.18 Forty-three-year-old man with a craniotomy for resection of a meningioma, prominent Mu rhythm over C3 in the setting of breach effect.

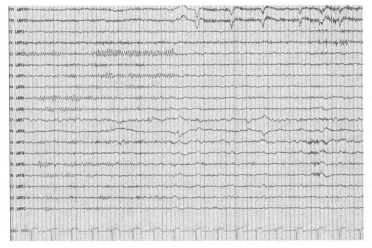

Figure 13.19 Same waveforms seen in Figure 13.18 in average reference montage.

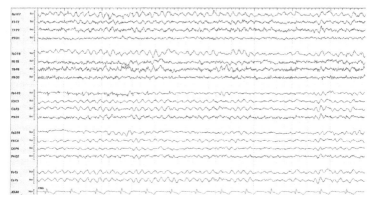

Figure 13.20 Thirty-three-year-old man with shaking spells, frontocentral theta during active smart phone use.

Posterior Variants

These are seen in the occipital channels and occur either as isolated waveforms or trains.

Positive Occipital Sharp Transients of Sleep (POSTS)

Appearance: Positive (downward) occipital sharp waves, often in trains, and commonly asymmetric in amplitude [4].

Location: occipital (phase reverse at O1 or O2)

State: drowsiness and early sleep

Age Group: adolescents and young adults

Clinical Caveat: Confirm positive polarity on a referential montage. Figure 13.21 shows POSTS in drowsiness. Figures 13.22 and 13.23 show POSTS in longitudinal and referential montage, respectively, note the positive deflection in the occipital channels on ear reference (Figure 13.23).

Lambda Waves

Appearance: Look like POSTS, but in wakefulness, and can also be asymmetric.

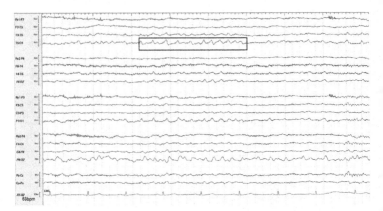

Figure 13.21 Forty-six-year-old man in light sleep, POSTs over the occipital channels.

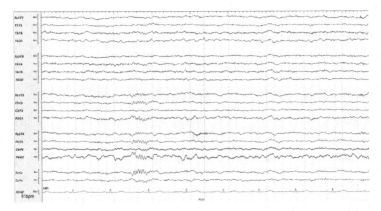

Figure 13.22 Forty-nine-year-old woman in sleep, POSTs in the occipital channels.

Location: occipital

State: wakefulness (active visual exploration)

Age Group: adolescents and young adults

Clinical Caveat: Seen during active visual exploration, hence commonly occur with lateral eye movements. Figure 13.24 shows lambda waves – note features

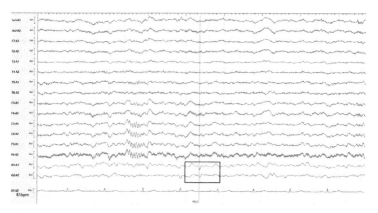

Figure 13.23 Same waveforms as in Figure 13.22 in ear reference; note the downward (positive) deflections definitive for this waveform.

of an "awake" background including eye blink artifact and a reactive posterior-dominant rhythm [6].

Posterior Slow Waves of Youth (PSWY)

Appearance: Often isolated intrusions of broad delta or theta waves (slowing) in the background alpha that are asymmetric and asynchronous [6].

Location: occipital or parietal

State: wakefulness

Age Group: children and young adults

Clinical Caveat: These are reactive to eye opening or alerting stimulation. They increase with hyperventilation. Figure 13.25 shows posterior slow waves of youth.

Notes

1. Some authors believe that occasional focal temporal delta slowing in asymptomatic adults over 60 years of age may be permissible in limited circumstances. *Benign temporal delta transients of the elderly* refers to occasional, small, single, rounded, or irregular delta waves that do not disturb an otherwise normal and symmetric background. These waves are attenuated during wakefulness and accentuated

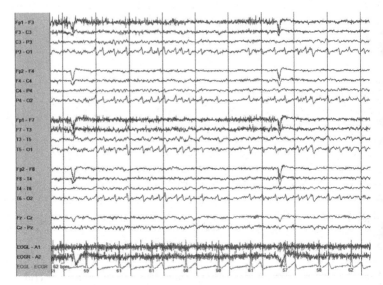

Figure 13.24 Twenty-eight-year-old woman during wakefulness, lambda waves in the occipital channels.

during drowsiness or hyperventilation. Their occurrence should be less than once per ten pages (<1% of the record). They may occur in pairs but never trains [7].

2. Antiepileptic medications such as valproic acid or levetiracetam may blunt epileptic discharges and reduce their amplitude, making them less distinct from the surrounding background, these blunted discharges can be mistaken for variants [8].

Chapter Summary

1. Benign variants should be distinguished from epileptogenic and ictal patterns to prevent misdiagnosis of epilepsy.
2. Variants are identified based on their appearance, typical location, state, and age group.
3. Antiepileptic medications such as valproic acid or levetiracetam may blunt epileptic discharges and reduce their amplitude, making them less distinct from the surrounding background. These can be mistaken for normal variants.

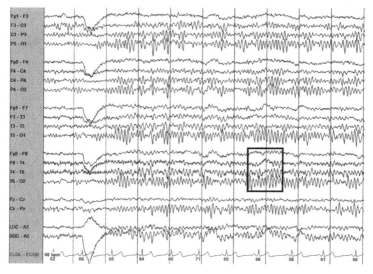

Figure 13.25 Seventeen-year-old girl during wakefulness, posterior slow waves of youth over the posterior temporal region.

Sharp Variants

Variant	Appearance	Location	State	Age group
Wickets	Clusters	Temporal	Drowsiness	Adults
SSS	Singles	Temporal	Drowsiness	Adults
14 and 6 Hz	Bursts	Temporal	Drowsiness	Children
Phantom spikes	Bursts	Diffuse	Drowsiness	Young

Rhythmic Variants

Variant	Frequency	Location	State	Age group
FAR	3–7 Hz	Frontal	Arousal	Children
RMTD	5–7 Hz	Midtemporal	Drowsiness	Adults
SREDA	5–7 Hz	Diffuse	Drowsiness	Adults (>50 years)
Midline theta	5–8 Hz	Midline	Drowsiness	Adults
Mu	8–13 Hz	Central	Awake	Young

Posterior Variants

Variant	Appearance	Location	State	Age group
POSTS	Positive sharps	Occipital	Sleep	Young
LAMBDA	Positive sharps	Occipital	Awake	Young
PSWY	Isolated slowing	Occipital	Awake	Young

References

1. Smith D, Defalla BA, Chadwick DW. The misdiagnosis of epilepsy and the management of refractory epilepsy in a specialist clinic. *QJM*. 1999 Jan 1;**92**(1):15–23.

2. Aminoff MJ. Electroencephalography: general principles and clinical applications. In *Electrodiagnosis in clinical neurology*, 6th ed.; Aminoff, MJ, Ed. (pp. 37–84). Elsevier, New York; 2012.

3. Krauss GL, Abdallah A, Lesser R, Thompson RE, Niedermeyer E. Clinical and EEG features of patients with EEG wicket rhythms misdiagnosed with epilepsy. *Neurology*. 2005 Jun 14;**64**(11):1879–83.

4. Tatum WO IV, Husain AM, Benbadis SR, et al. Normal adult EEG and patterns of uncertain significance. *Journal of Clinical Neurophysiology*. 2006;**23**(3):194–207.

5. Tatum WO, DiCiaccio B, Kipta JA, Yelvington KH, Stein MA. The texting rhythm: a novel EEG waveform using smartphones. *Journal of Clinical Neurophysiology*. 2016 Aug 1;**33**(4):359–66.

6. Aird RB, Gastaut Y. Occipital and posterior electroencephalographic ryhthms. *Electroencephalography and Clinical Neurophysiology*. 1959 Nov 1;**11**(4):637–56.

7. Van Cott AC. Epilepsy and EEG in the elderly. *Epilepsia*. 2002 Mar; **43**:94–102.

8. Libenson MH, Caravale B. Do antiepileptic drugs differ in suppressing interictal epileptiform activity in children? *Pediatric Neurology*. 2001 Mar 1;**24**(3):214–18.

Sporadic Abnormalities

Sporadic abnormalities are those that occur in singles, sometimes in pairs or in abundance, but they aren't repetitive (i.e., do not reappear in quick succession or after fixed intervals).

Sporadic abnormalities indicate underlying cortical dysfunction, though an associated structural lesion may not be always evident on neuroimaging (it should be sought) [1].

Three principal points of information are to be gained from the identification of sporadic abnormalities. These are as follows:

1. Where is the problem (i.e., location of the dysfunction)?
2. What is the problem (i.e., hint of potential etiology)?
3. Is there a predilection for epileptic seizures (i.e., epileptogenicity)?

The EEG cannot localize a lesion with the precision of modern neuroimaging techniques and electrographic abnormalities are notoriously nonspecific to etiology (only suggestive at best). The key role of the reader is to determine if an abnormality suggests a predilection for experiencing or developing epileptic seizures (epileptogenicity) as this determines the need for antiepileptic therapy [1].

"Sharpness" of the waveform at its peak (shape) is the main electrographic feature based on which this determination is made, the other being immediate surrounding activity.

Specifically look at the peak of the predominant phase of the discharge (the phase with the greatest amplitude), then measure its duration at the baseline. If the duration of the phase is less than 200 ms at baseline, categorize it as a *potentially* epileptiform abnormality (spike or sharp wave). The rest are slow waves. Slow waves with sharp peaks may be called "sharply contoured" but these do not qualify as spike or sharp waves [2].

Therefore, based on the sharpness of their peak and duration at baseline, sporadic abnormalities may be classified into two types:

1. spikes and sharp waves
2. slow waves

Figure 14.1 shows the key differences between spikes, sharp waves, and slow waves.

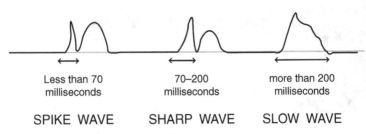

Less than 70 milliseconds

70–200 milliseconds

more than 200 milliseconds

SPIKE WAVE   SHARP WAVE   SLOW WAVE

Figure 14.1 Types of sporadic abnormalities.

Spike and Sharp Waves

Spike and sharp waves have pointed peaks and are both epileptiform abnormalities or epileptic discharges. These are waveforms (or complexes, i.e., combination of waves), associated with a predisposition to experiencing epileptic seizures. It is important to understand that the mere presence of a spike or sharp wave is not pathognomic for epilepsy, it only means that there is a strong likelihood of experiencing an epileptic seizure. Conversely, a very small percentage of healthy people will have spike or sharp waves on their EEG [3].

Conventionally, spikes last more than 20 ms and less than 70 ms, while sharp waves last more than 70 ms but less than 200 ms (Figure 14.1). These are often followed by slow waves and together form a spike/sharp and slow-wave complex (called spike waves or sharp waves for short).

Sometimes there may be more than one spike in a complex, these are called polyspikes (Figure 14.2).

The terms spike and sharp waves may be used interchangeably and essentially mean the same thing – a predisposition to epileptic seizures. Often, both occur in the same disorder or the same patient.

Based on sharpness alone, many different waveforms including benign variants and artifacts may also resemble spike or sharp waves. When you suspect a spike or sharp wave, the next step is to confirm it as an epileptic discharge based on a few key electrographic features. We described these features in Chapter 13 for sharp variants. Let's revisit them again in the context of a spike or sharp wave.

Three key features on an epileptic discharge are as follows:

1. *Disruption of background activities:* Look at the immediate surrounding activity, before and after the discharge, epileptic discharges not only have a higher amplitude compared to the surrounding background activity but appear to disrupt it.
2. *Aftercoming slow wave:* Often, epileptic discharges will be followed by a negative slow wave of 150–350 ms duration and variable amplitude.

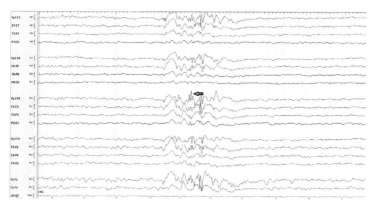

Figure 14.2 Twenty-three-year-old man with JME, frontal-predominant generalized polyspikes.

This may represent prolonged hyperpolarization due to secondary inhibition of a large neuronal population.

3. *Physiological field:* Epileptic discharges, as other forms of cerebral activity have physiological fields, this helps differentiate them from artifacts.

Other Features

- *Asymmetrical slopes:* The main component of the discharge has asymmetrical slopes with the first deflection being steepest.
- *Negative polarity:* The main component of the discharge is pointing upward. Rarely, positive spikes occur where the main component is positive (pointing downward); these may be seen after brain surgery, in neonates with periventricular hemorrhage or leukomalacia and children with multifocal epilepsies.
- Drops below the baseline.
- *Polyphasic:* crosses the baseline multiple times.
- Enhanced by drowsiness and non–rapid eye movement sleep [4].

Sharp waves that do not meet the criteria for a discharge may be called "sharp transients." Figure 14.3 demonstrates the typical features of an epileptic discharge and Figure 14.4 shows positive spikes.

Once confirmed to be epileptic discharges, they can be further categorized based on their location:

1. focal
2. generalized

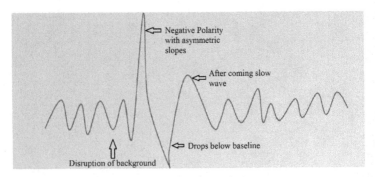

Figure 14.3 Features of an epileptic discharge.

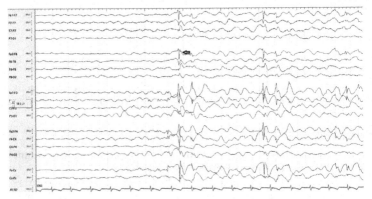

Figure 14.4 Seven-year-old boy with epilepsy, positive (downward) spikes.

Focal Discharges

Focal discharges originate from a single hemisphere and usually occur over a specific region. They may indicate focal epilepsy. If these occur independently over multiple regions, they are called multifocal discharges. The specific location of the focal discharge determines the strength of the association with focal epilepsy.

The strength of association with epilepsy is greatest for temporal and frontal discharges compared to other locations such as the centrotemporal (Rolandic), central, parietal, and occipital locations. For example, about 90% of those with anterior temporal spikes will have epilepsy compared to about

38% of those with Rolandic spikes. Approximately 60% of children with occipital spikes do not have epilepsy [5]. Occipital spikes are also common in nonepileptic conditions such as migraines and congenital blindness [6,7]. Approximately 94% of those with multifocal spikes have epileptic seizures [8]. Figure 14.5 shows a focal sharp wave (left temporal), and Figure 14.6 shows a focal spike wave (right temporal).

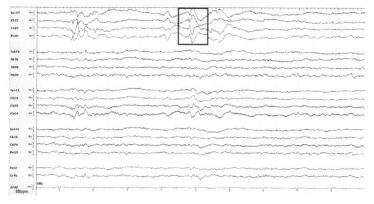

Figure 14.5 Fifty-year-old man with focal onset epilepsy, left temporal (T7) sharps.

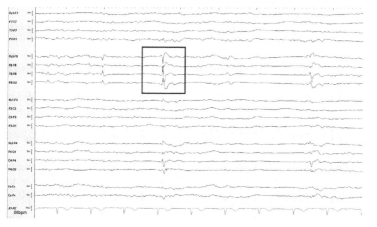

Figure 14.6 Sixty-seven-year-old woman with a stroke, right temporal (T8) spikes.

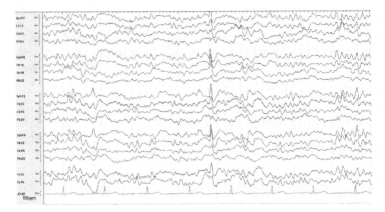

Figure 14.7 Thirty-one-year-old woman with LGS, frontal-predominant generalized sharps.

Generalized Discharges

These discharges originate simultaneously over both hemispheres, often maximal over the frontal regions and indicate generalized epilepsies. They may occur in singles, but more often in bursts of 1–3 s and can be longer. Longer runs (generalized spike waves) are typically associated with a subtle interference in mental function (absences). The frequency of the discharges determines the association with specific generalized epilepsies. Figure 14.7 shows a generalized sharp wave, Figure 14.8 shows a generalized spike wave.

Generalized spike and wave discharges (GSW) of approximately 2.5 to 3 Hz in frequency are the electrographic hallmark of typical absence seizures that occur in childhood absence epilepsy (Figure 14.9) [9].

Faster GSWs of approximately 4 to 6 Hz are seen with other generalized epilepsies such as juvenile myoclonic epilepsy (JME) and juvenile absence epilepsy (JAE), as shown in Figure 14.10 [10].

Slower GSWs of approximately 1.5 to 2.5 Hz are seen with Lennox–Gastaut syndrome (LGS) as shown in Figure 14.11 [11].

Generalized discharges may be activated or enhanced by photic stimulation and hyperventilation. Focal appearing or asymmetric fragments of generalized discharges are also common in those with generalized epilepsies [10].

Focal Discharges That Appear Generalized: In some acquired epilepsies such as posttraumatic epilepsy, focal discharges, particularly of frontal onset, can

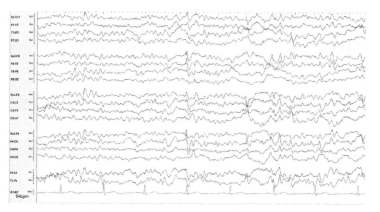

Figure 14.8 Same patient as in Figure 14.7, frontal-predominant generalized spikes.

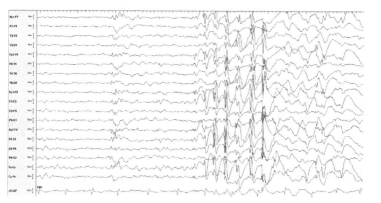

Figure 14.9 Eight-year-old boy with CAE, 3 Hz GSW discharges.

appear generalized. This happens when a focal or regional discharge directly leads to a corresponding contralateral discharge (bi-synchronous spike/sharp waves), this phenomenon is called as secondary bilateral synchrony. Another common situation occurs when a focal or regional discharge has a wide field that extends to the contralateral hemisphere, falsely appearing generalized.

Using a transverse montage, it is possible to distinguish such a wide field (large generator) from two discrete bi-synchronous generators. Often, other

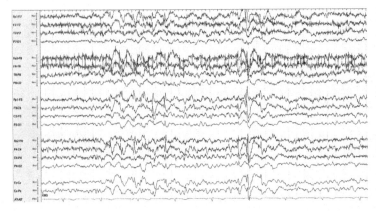

Figure 14.10 Seventeen-year-old boy with JME, 4 Hz GSW discharges.

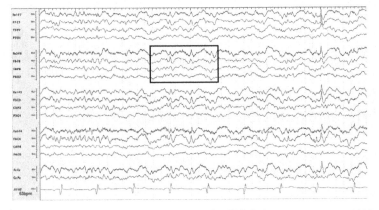

Figure 14.11 Same patient as in Figure 14.7, 2 Hz GSW discharges.

ipsilateral focal abnormalities such as slowing also suggest a focal rather than a true generalized discharge. Rarely, two distinct generators may occur in the same hemisphere to produce asynchronous focal discharges. Figure 14.12 demonstrates the difference between a generalized discharge, a focal discharge with a wide field and focal discharge with secondary bilateral synchrony. Figure 14.13 shows focal (right frontotemporal) discharges with wide contralateral fields that appear generalized.

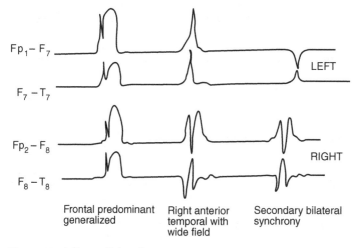

$Fp_1 - F_7$

$F_7 - T_7$

LEFT

$Fp_2 - F_8$

$F_8 - T_8$

RIGHT

Frontal predominant generalized

Right anterior temporal with wide field

Secondary bilateral synchrony

Figure 14.12 Types of bilateral appearing discharges.

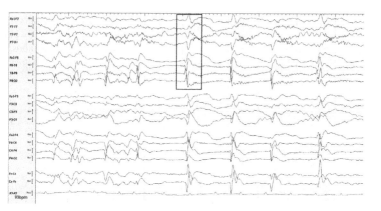

Figure 14.13 Same patient as in Figure 14.6, right temporal discharges (T8) with wide fields.

Slow Waves

Slowing is the presence of abnormal delta or theta (slow) waves. Normal slow waves (physiological slowing) is seen in drowsiness or sleep and is described in Chapter 8.

"Delta slowing" was so named by W. G. Walter, its discoverer, because of its association with the three "Ds" of disease, degeneration, and death. Its presence indicates underlying cerebral dysfunction. Often multiple types of slowing coexist in a single record. Slowing by itself is typically not associated with epileptic seizures, though temporal-predominant lateralized rhythmic delta activity (previously called Temporal Intermittent Rhythmic Delta or TIRDA) is an important exception [12].

As with all foreground abnormalities, slowing should be described based on three key features:

1. location (focal, bi-hemispheric, generalized, or multifocal)
2. occurrence (sporadic or repetitive; see the following chapter)
3. morphology (polymorphic or monomorphic)

In addition, the constituent frequency of the slow waves (theta, delta, or mixed theta-delta waves) and reactivity to stimuli or drowsiness should also be noted. Further modifiers include the prevalence (continuous or intermittent), duration, amplitude, and frequency as described in Chapter 12.

Figure 14.14 shows intermittent left temporal (focal) polymorphic slowing, Figure 14.15 shows continuous left hemispheric (focal) polymorphic slowing and Figure 14.16 shows intermittent left temporal (focal) monomorphic slowing.

Bi-hemispheric (bilateral) slowing should be differentiated from generalized or diffuse slowing. Bi-hemispheric slowing, like generalized slowing appears in both hemispheres however it is typically not symmetric or synchronous. Generalized rhythmic slowing is further discussed in the following chapter (Chapter 15).

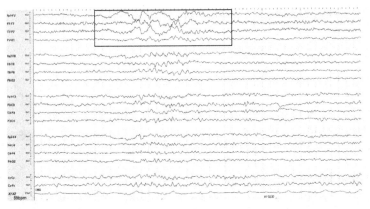

Figure 14.14 Sixty-two-year-old lady with a first-time seizure, intermittent focal left temporal polymorphic slowing.

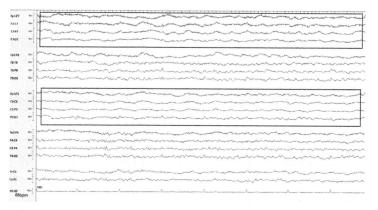

Figure 14.15 Sixty-eight-year-old man with a left hemispheric stroke, continuous left hemispheric polymorphic delta slowing.

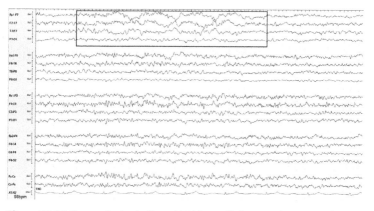

Figure 14.16 Same patient as in Figure 14.14, burst of left temporal monomorphic slowing.

Figure 14.17 shows intermittent bitemporal, but left>right polymorphic slowing, Figure 14.18 shows intermittent bursts of generalized slowing and Figure 14.19 shows continuous bi-hemispheric (bilateral) but left>right polymorphic slowing.

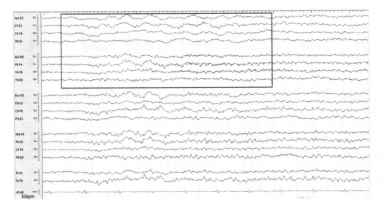

Figure 14.17 Eighty-two-year-old man with delirium, left greater than right bitemporal polymorphic delta slowing.

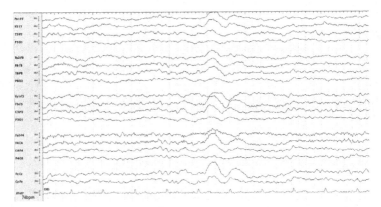

Figure 14.18 Same patient as in Figure 14.17, intermittent brief burst of generalized delta slowing.

Clinical Correlation

1. Generalized slowing diffusely affects both cerebral hemispheres, bi-hemispheric slowing is bilateral but affects each hemisphere in unequal measures, hence unlike generalized slowing, bi-hemispheric slowing is typically asynchronous and asymmetric.

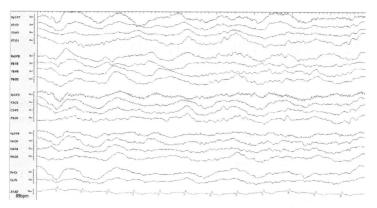

Figure 14.19 Seventy-year-old man with coma, continuous bi-hemispheric delta slowing.

2. Polymorphic slowing is a nonspecific sign of cerebral dysfunction, when focal, it suggests a localization.

3. Monomorphic (rhythmic) slowing may indicate epileptogenicity; more on this in the following chapter.

4. Continuous slowing may indicate static dysfunction (e.g., stroke or tumor), while intermittent slowing may be indicative of fluctuating dysfunction (e.g., postictal, migraines, transient hypoperfusion, or delirium).

5. Lower frequencies, higher amplitudes, and greater prevalence may correspond to the severity of dysfunction. A reversal of these features over time could be indicative of electrographic improvement.

6. Neither of the above features are sensitive or specific to the severity or etiology of the dysfunction.

Chapter Summary

1. Sporadic abnormalities are those that occur in singles, in pairs, or in abundance but are not repetitive.

2. They indicate cortical dysfunction, but the central question is epileptogenicity.

3. The key electrographic feature to classify the waveform is its sharpness.

4. Spike and sharp waves are pointed in morphology and are typically epileptogenic; these terms are often used interchangeably.

5. Slow waves are blunted in morphology and are typically not epileptogenic (except rhythmic focal slowing).

6. Spikes are 20 to 70 ms and sharp waves are 70–200 ms in duration; anything greater than 200 ms is a slow wave. Though spikes appear sharper/ more pointed than sharp waves, they essentially mean the same thing – an association with epileptic seizures (not pathognomic for epilepsy).

7. Three key features of an epileptic discharge (sharp or spike wave) are its disruption of the normal background, an aftercoming slow wave and a physiological field.

8. Based on their location, epileptic discharges may be classified as focal (one hemisphere), generalized (both hemispheres), bi-hemispheric (both hemispheres but asynchronous), and multifocal.

9. The specific location of the focal discharge determines the strength of its association with focal epilepsy.

10. The frequency of the generalized discharge determines the specific association with generalized epilepsies.

11. Sometimes a focal discharge may appear generalized, as in secondary bilateral synchrony (two synchronous generators), or with a wide field (single large generator). A transverse montage helps distinguish these.

12. Sporadic slowing should be described based on its location (generalized, bi-hemispheric, focal, or multifocal) and morphology (monomorphic or polymorphic). It may be continuous or intermittent.

13. Polymorphic slowing is a nonspecific marker of cerebral dysfunction; monomorphic (rhythmic) slowing may indicate epileptogenicity.

14. Continuous slowing is indicative of static cortical dysfunction (e.g., stroke), while intermittent slowing may indicate fluctuating (dynamic) cortical dysfunction (e.g., postictal).

15. Electrographic features of slowing are neither sensitive nor specific to the severity/etiology of cerebral dysfunction. Slowing merely indicates the presence of cerebral dysfunction and in specific circumstances – epileptogenicity.

References

1. King MA, Newton MR, Jackson GD, et al. Epileptology of the first-seizure presentation: a clinical, electroencephalographic, and magnetic resonance imaging study of 300 consecutive patients. *The Lancet*. 1998 Sep 26;352(9133):1007–11.

2. Hirsch LJ, LaRoche SM, Gaspard N, et al. American clinical neurophysiology society's standardized critical care EEG terminology: 2012 version. *Journal of Clinical Neurophysiology*. 2013 Feb 1;**30**(1):1–27.

3. Sam MC, So EL. Significance of epileptiform discharges in patients without epilepsy in the community. *Epilepsia*. 2001 Oct 29;**42**(10):1273–8.

4. Niedermeyer E. Abnormal EEG patterns: epileptic and paroxysmal. In Electroencephalography: basic principles, clinical applications, and related fields (p. 255). Oxford University Press, Oxford; 2005.

5. Fois A, Malandrini F, Tomaccini D. Clinical findings in children with occipital paroxysmal discharges. *Epilepsia*. 1988 Oct;**29**(5):620–3.

6. Slatter KH. Some clinical and EEG findings in patients with migraine. *Brain*. 1968 Mar 1;**91**(1):85–98.

7. Kellaway P, Bloxsom A, MacGregor M. Occipital spike foci associated with retro-lental fibroplasia and other forms of retinal loss in children. *Electroencephalography and Clinical Neurophysiology*. 1955 Jan 1;**7**(3):469–70.

8. Pedley TA. Interictal epileptiform discharges: discriminating characteristics and clinical correlations. *American Journal of EEG Technology*. 1980 Sep 1;**20**(3):101–19.

9. Hedström A, Olsson I. Epidemiology of absence epilepsy: EEG findings and their predictive value. *Pediatric Neurology*. 1991 Mar 1;**7**(2):100–4.

10. Seneviratne U, Hepworth G, Cook M, D'Souza W. Atypical EEG abnormalities in genetic generalized epilepsies. *Clinical Neurophysiology*. 2016 Jan 1;**127**(1):214–20.

11. Ferlazzo E, Nikaronova M, Italiano D, et al. Lennox–Gastaut syndrome in adulthood: clinical and EEG features. *Epilepsy Research*. 2010 May 1;**89**(2):271–7.

12. Bazil CW, Herman ST, Pedley TA. Focal electroencephalographic abnormalities. In *Current practice of clinical electroencephalography* (pp. 303–47). Lippincott Williams and Wilkins, New York; 2003.

Repetitive Abnormalities

These are abnormal waveforms with relative uniform morphology that repeat either in rapid succession (rhythmic), after nearly regular intervals (periodic) or as recurring spike or sharp and slow waves (spike and wave). The pattern must continue for at least six cycles (six times) to qualify as a repetitive abnormality [1].

Therefore, repetitive abnormalities may be one of three types:

1. periodic;
2. rhythmic;
3. spike and wave.

Figure 15.1 shows sporadic and repetitive abnormalities.

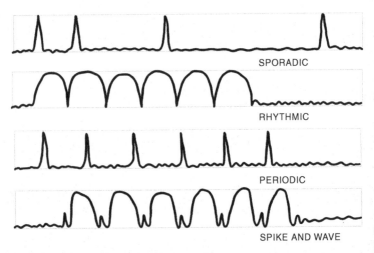

SPORADIC

RHYTHMIC

PERIODIC

SPIKE AND WAVE

Figure 15.1 Sporadic and repetitive abnormalities.

Repetitive abnormalities are common in critically ill patients and, like sporadic abnormalities, represent underlying cortical dysfunction. Periodic patterns are also markers of neuronal injury, independently predicting poor outcomes [1,2]. All repetitive abnormalities can be associated with epileptic seizures (epileptogenic); the strength of this association varies by abnormality. The association is maximum with lateralized periodic discharges (LPDs); it is also high with lateralized rhythmic delta activity (LRDA) and generalized periodic discharges (GPDs) but least with generalized rhythmic delta activity (GRDA). However, unlike sporadic abnormalities, repetitive abnormalities in specific situations may themselves represent the electrographic seizure activity, and these are called ictal patterns. This implies that repetitive abnormalities lie on an ictal–interictal continuum. An epileptogenic (interictal) pattern may evolve into an electrographic seizure (ictal pattern) and vice versa in the same patient during the same or subsequent recording. Therefore, determining the ictal potential of a repetitive pattern is crucial to its management [1,2,3]. Ictal patterns are described further in Chapter 16.

This chapter instructs the reader on how to correctly describe repetitive patterns based on standardized critical care EEG terminology proposed by the American Clinical Neurophysiology Society (ACNS) [1]. In the later part of this chapter, commonly encountered repetitive patterns are described along with potential ictal characteristics.

According to standardized terminology, the reader **should describe** each pattern as a combination of two main terms (main term 1 and main term 2). Subsequently, other descriptors, such as prevalence, duration, frequency, phases, sharpness, amplitude, and polarity, may be added to this combination. There is excellent interrater agreement on these main terms [1].

Main Term 1

Generalized (G). When a pattern equally involves both hemispheres, it is called a "generalized" pattern. It may show frontal, occipital, or central predominance based on its maximal amplitude in a referential montage.

Lateralized (L). When a pattern is prominent over one hemisphere, it is called a "lateralized" pattern. A lateralized pattern may have a focal or regional field, or it may be bilateral with a wide field but is clearly predominant over a single hemisphere.

When two distinct patterns of the same repetitive abnormality occur asynchronously, there are called independent patterns (I). The term *bilateral independent* (BI) is used when they occur bilaterally, and *unilateral independent* (UI) when they occur in the same hemisphere. The main term *multifocal*

(Mf) is used to describe more than two distinct patterns of the same repetitive abnormality.

Main Term 2

Periodic Discharges (PD): These are repeating epileptic discharges with uniform morphologies that reappear at regular intervals. The reader should distinguish a discharge from a burst. Bursts have multiple phases (polyphasic) and longer durations (at least more than half a second).

Rhythmic Delta Activity (RDA): These are repeating monomorphic delta waves that recur uninterrupted, that is, without intervals between the consecutive waves.

Spike and Wave (SW): These are spike or sharp waves (or polyspikes) that are consistently followed by slow waves in a regular repeating run. Each spike or sharp wave is always followed by a slow wave such as a spike and wave, polyspikes and wave, or sharp and wave.

After you have closely inspected the repetitive pattern, choose an appropriate main term 1 and combine it with the appropriate main term 2 to describe the waveform. Example: A generalized periodic pattern would be called generalized (main term 1) periodic discharges (main term 2) or GPD for short.

If you think a pattern qualifies as both periodic and rhythmic, it should be coded as periodic with a rhythmic plus term (+R). A plus term renders the pattern ictal in appearance and is described in detail in Chapter 16.

All repetitive patterns including ictal patterns (seizures) may be induced by stimulation. The term *SI* is added before the combination of main terms to describe a stimulus induced pattern (e.g., SI-GPDs for stimulus-induced GPDs). The inducing stimulus should also be specified (example: suctioning). Stimulus-induced rhythmic, periodic, or ictal discharges (previously called SIRPIDs) are common in critically ill patients, but their true pathologic, prognostic, or therapeutic significance is not known [4]. Figure 15.2 shows a stimulus-induced GRDA (SI-GRDA).

Common Repetitive Abnormalities

Though many combinations of main terms 1 and 2 exist, the following abnormalities are commonly encountered in clinical practice:

Rhythmic Patterns
- generalized – rhythmic delta activity (GRDA)
- lateralized – rhythmic delta activity (LRDA)

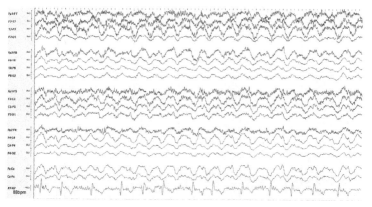

Figure 15.2 Eighty-three-year-old woman with dementia complicated by a urinary tract infection, stimulus-induced 2–3 Hz GRDA with tactile stimulation. There is prominent muscle artifact over the left hemispheric channels associated with arousal.

Periodic Patterns

- generalized – periodic discharges (GPD)
- generalized periodic discharges with triphasic morphology (triphasic waves)
- lateralized – periodic discharges (LPD)
- bilateral independent – periodic discharges (BIPD)

Spike and Wave Patterns

- generalized spike and wave (GSW)

Generalized Rhythmic Delta Activity (GRDA)

This is a diffuse, high-amplitude, monomorphic rhythmic delta activity that is commonly seen in encephalopathic patients. The pattern may be stimulus induced or associated with a state change (arousal) and is least associated with seizures. There are two common subtypes:

Frontally Predominant GRDA (Common in Adults): This was previously called frontal intermittent rhythmic delta activity (FIRDA). This pattern is nonspecific for etiology and is least associated with epileptic seizures. It is most commonly associated with toxic or metabolic encephalopathies, although it can also be seen with structural brain lesions or raised intracranial pressure [5]. Figure 15.3 shows frontally predominant GRDA.

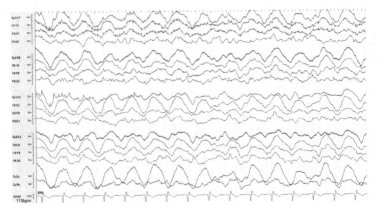

Figure 15.3 Sixty-five-year-old man with sepsis, frontally predominant 1.5–2 Hz GRDA.

Occipitally Predominant GRDA (Common in Children): This was previously called occipital intermittent rhythmic delta activity (OIRDA) and is a nonspecific pattern, but rarely it is associated generalized epilepsies (epileptogenic), particularly childhood absence epilepsy (CAE). It is more commonly associated with a toxic metabolic encephalopathy, structural brain lesions, or raised intracranial pressure [6]. Figure 23.3 (Chapter 23) shows occipital predominant GRDA (or OIRDA) in a patient with childhood absence epilepsy (CAE).

Lateralized Rhythmic Delta Activity (LRDA)

This is a focal monomorphic, often sharply contoured, rhythmic delta slowing that occurs in short bursts of a few seconds but may be longer in encephalopathic patients. The pattern is most commonly predominant over the temporal region but is not restricted to it. LRDA is independently associated with epileptic seizures (epileptogenic). Focal abnormalities such as LPDs often coexist. Typically, an underlying acute or remote structural lesion is present [7]. Temporal intermittent rhythmic delta activity (TIRDA) is a subtype of LRDA that is seen in patients with mesial temporal lobe epilepsy, typically seen in the ambulatory setting [8]. Figure 15.4 shows left frontal–predominant LRDA, whereas Figure 20.2 (Chapter 20) shows left temporal intermittent rhythmic delta activity (TIRDA).

Generalized Periodic Discharges (GPD)

These are diffuse, usually symmetric, periodic discharges. They may show frontal or occipital predominance. They were previously called generalized

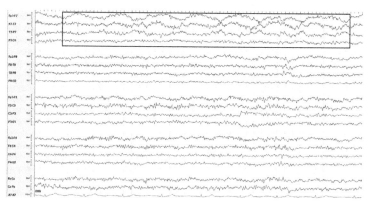

Figure 15.4 Sixty-two-year-old woman with a first-time seizure, 1 Hz left frontal–predominant LRDA.

periodic epileptiform discharges (GPEDs), but the word *epileptiform* has since been removed as they may not always be associated with seizures (e.g., nonictal triphasic waves) and their morphology isn't always epileptiform. GPDs may be stimulus induced (SI-GPDs) or associated with a change of state (e.g., arousals). In specific situations, GPDs may represent the electrographic manifestation of electrographic seizures and therefore constitute an ictal pattern.

GPDs are commonly seen in the following conditions:

1. toxic or metabolic encephalopathies, including sepsis (esp. triphasic waves);
2. extensive structural cerebral damage such as hypoxic ischemic encephalopathy, diffuse intracranial hemorrhage, or neurodegeneration;
3. epileptic encephalopathies;
4. medications such as cefepime, Lithium, Ifosfamide, Baclofen, or Metrizamide;
5. infections such as Creutzfeldt–Jakob disease (CJD) or subacute sclerosing panencephalitis (SSPE).

GPDs are traditionally thought to imply poor prognosis, however, recent studies have not found an independent association with increased mortality. GPDs have been associated with nonconvulsive status epilepticus (NCSE), which is itself associated with increased mortality. The underlying etiology and severity of the primary disease process are most often the key determinants of prognosis in these patients [9,10]. Figure 15.5 shows occipital-predominant GPDs.

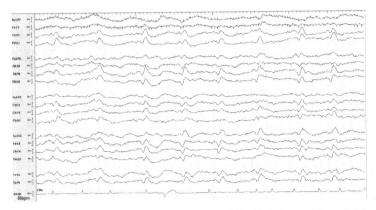

Figure 15.5 Seventy-five-year-old man with Creutzfeldt–Jakob disease, 1 Hz occipital-predominant GPDs.

Generalized Periodic Discharges with Triphasic Morphology (Triphasic Waves)

This is a common subtype of GPDs that is encountered in patients with toxic or metabolic encephalopathies (such as hepatic or uremic encephalopathies) but may also be seen with multiple different etiologies including hypoxic and epileptic encephalopathies. Less commonly, triphasic waves may be the electrographic manifestation of NCSE. These ictal triphasic waves can be distinguished from nonictal triphasic waves based on electrographic features and a response to trials of benzodiazepines or nonsedating antiepileptic medications such as levetiracetam [11].

Triphasic waves (TW) are identified on EEG using two key features:

1. Triphasic waves often have two baseline crossings or three phases. "Phases" are determined by the number of baseline crossings seen in a typical discharge in longitudinal bipolar montage. Look at the channel in which the discharge is best appreciated. A triphasic wave will typically cross the baseline twice, each of the three phases is longer than the previous and may be negative (up)-positive(down)-negative(up). The positive phase (down/phase II) is typically of highest amplitude. Sometimes, the initial negative phase is not clearly seen and only a prominent positive (down) and negative (up) phase are seen, these bi-phasic waves (phases II–III only) may also be categorized as triphasic waves [1].

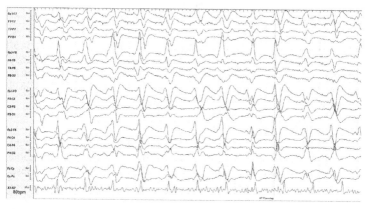

Figure 15.6 Seventy-seven-year-old man with sepsis on cefepime, 1–2 Hz triphasic waves with prominent AP phase lag.

2. Triphasic waves often have an anterior–posterior or posterior-anterior lag. This applies if a consistent measurable delay of more than 100 ms exists from the anterior most channel to the posterior most channel in which the wave is seen or vice versa (posterior-anterior lag). You should use both a longitudinal and a referential montage (ipsilateral ear reference) to evaluate lag [1]. Figure 15.6 shows generalized periodic discharges with triphasic morphology (triphasic waves).

After you have identified triphasic waves, the next step is to estimate if they are potentially ictal. This can be done based on electrographic features and a response to anti-epileptic medication trial.

Electrographic Features

Electrographic features suggestive of potentially nonictal triphasic include the following:

- presence of a phase lag;
- dominant phase II (down);
- longer duration of phase I (not a sharp/spike);
- slower frequencies;
- stimulus induction or with arousal from drowsiness/sleep (state dependency).

Features suggestive of potentially ictal triphasic include the following:

- overriding spikes or sharp waves;
- faster frequencies (>2.5 Hz);
- no change in the pattern with state change or stimulation.

However, it must be noted that no specific electrographic features have been identified that either alone or in combination can reliably distinguish triphasic waves that respond to treatment (presumably ictal) vs. those that do not (presumably nonictal). Therefore, experts have proposed a trial of anticonvulsant medications in cases of incompletely explained encephalopathies with triphasic waves. Based on a single retrospective study, almost one-third of all "metabolic" triphasic waves may show a definitive response to medication [11,12].

Anti-epileptic Medications Trial

Ictal triphasic waves are thought to respond to anti-epileptic medications (responders). Trials of low-dose benzodiazepines or a nonbenzodiazepine anti-epileptics (e.g., levetiracetam) may be used to evaluate for a response. Typically, the patient is monitored at least for 24–48 hours with continuous electroencephalography during the trial.

Low-Dose Benzodiazepine Trial

One method is to administer small doses of lorazepam (up to 4 mg in divided doses of 1 mg each) with repeated clinical and EEG assessment before the first dose and after each subsequent dose. A successful trial is defined as the resolution of the triphasic waves AND either clear clinical improvement or appearance of previously absent normal EEG patterns (e.g., posterior-dominant rhythm). Mere resolution of the EEG without clinical improvement is considered an equivocal response. Most responses occur immediately (within 2 hours of initiating lorazepam), but late responders have also been described. Further doses of lorazepam should not be administered in the setting of hypotension or respiratory depression [11,12].

Levetiracetam Trial

Recent studies have shown a greater response rate of triphasic waves to non benzodiazepines anti-epileptics (most commonly levetiracetam), compared to benzodiazepines, suggesting this to be a useful strategy even in those with an inconclusive response to benzodiazepines. Late responses were also common (greater than 2 hours after initiating the trial). A loading dose of levetiracetam (25 mg/kg as a single intravenous dose) followed by maintenance dosing of 1.5 gram twice daily for 48 hours is typically used in our practice. Success of the trial is defined in the same way as for lorazepam that is, resolution of the triphasic waves AND either definite clinical improvement or emergence of previously absent normal patterns such as a posterior dominant rhythm. Other less sedating antiepileptics may also be used in place of levetiracetam [11,12,13]. Figure 15.7 shows apparent ictal triphasic waves.

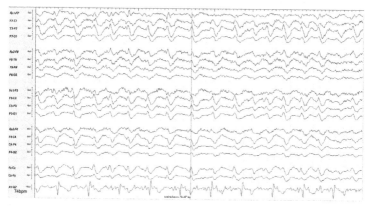

Figure 15.7 Same patient as in Figure 15.3, 2–2.5 Hz triphasic waves without AP phase lag.

Lateralized Periodic Discharges (LPD)

These are focal periodic patterns, lateralized to a single hemisphere (sometimes with wide fields). Previously, they were called periodic lateralized epileptiform discharges (PLEDs). They commonly lie close to the ictal end of the ictal–interictal continuum and in specific cases represent an ictal pattern. LPDs represent an underlying acute destructive cortical process that may not always be evident on neuroimaging. They appear within the first few days of injury and usually resolve in a few weeks. Chronic LPDs suggest the development of focal epilepsy. All forms of structural damage may cause LPDs; strokes, viral encephalitis, and hypoxic injury being the most common etiologies. LPDs are strongly associated with epileptic seizures (as high as 60% per some studies) [14,15]. Focal motor seizures being the commonest seizure type [14]. Seizures may appear late and they may not be convulsive. Therefore, continuous EEG monitoring for 24–72 hours should be considered in those with LPDs [16]. LPDs are also an independent risk factor for poor outcome in those with SAH and ICH [17,18]. Figure 15.8 shows right hemispheric LPDs.

After you have identified LPDs, the next step is to determine if they are ictal. Ictal LPDs can be distinguished from interictal LPDs based on their clinical correlates and electrographic features [19]:

Common Clinical Correlates of Ictal LPDs

1. *Focal clonic seizures (or epilepsia partialis continua):* Focal seizures or status epilepticus may be seen contralateral to the LPDs. Often, the

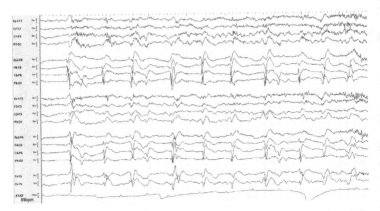

Figure 15.8 Seventy-two-year-old lady with HSV encephalitis, right hemispheric LPDs.

individual discharges are time locked to the EMG recording or myogenic artifact.

2. Subtle bedside clinical signs such as eye deviation, aphasia, hemiparesis,
hemianopia, sensory changes, or confusion may be associated with LPDs
located over eloquent areas such as fronto-polar, temporo-parietal and occipital regions. In these cases, a resolution of the LPDs in addition to clinical
improvement (focal symptoms or encephalopathy) in response to a low dose
of lorazepam or loading dose of antiepileptic medication may suggest ictal
LPDs. Further escalation of antiepileptic therapy may be necessary.

3. Some experts have suggested that evidence of regional hypermetabolism
such as an increased signal on PET or SPECT imaging with LPDs supports
an ictal pattern and warrants aggressive treatment [20].

The electrographic features of ictal LPDs are described later in Chapter 16.

Bilateral Independent Periodic Discharges (BIPD)

These are bilateral, independent, often asynchronous periodic discharges.
They are less common compared to LPDs but with similar etiology. They
are also thought to be associated with an increased seizure risk and are often
associated with severe encephalopathy [21]. Figure 15.9 shows BIPDs that
evolve into a seizure.

Generalized Spike and Wave (GSW)

Repetitive generalized spike and wave (GSW) discharges are epileptiform
patterns, and those occurring in runs of greater than 2.5 Hz are potentially

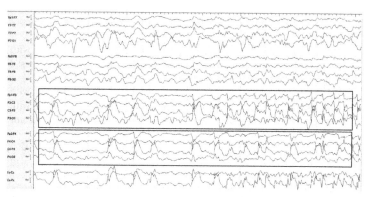

Figure 15.9 Sixty-year-old man with hepatic coma, BIPDs (central predominant) that evolve into an electrographic seizure over the left paracentral region.

ictal. Complexes may be composed of polyspikes/sharps and waves [1]. These patterns are further described in Chapter 16.

Chapter Summary

1. Repetitive waveforms may repeat in quick succession (rhythmic), after nearly regular intervals (periodic), or as spike and wave (SW).
2. Periodic discharges are considered markers for neuronal injury.
3. Repetitive abnormalities are epileptogenic, but the strength of their association with seizures is variable; in specific situations they may also represent ongoing electrographic seizures (ictal patterns).
4. A repetitive pattern is described as a combination of a main term 1 with a main term 2 based on the American Clinical Neurophysiology Society (ACNS) standardized critical care EEG terminology.
5. Main term 1 could be either generalized (G), lateralized (L), bilateral or unilaterally independent (BI or UI), or multifocal (Mf).
6. Main term 2 could be either periodic discharges (PD), rhythmic delta activity (RDA), or spike and wave (SW).
7. Common rhythmic abnormalities include GRDA and LRDA. Common periodic abnormalities include GPDs, LPDs, and BIPDs.
8. The term *SI* is added to the combination of main terms to denote a stimulus-induced pattern (e.g., SI-GPDs for stimulus-induced GPDs).
9. Frontal-predominant GRDA are most commonly seen in adults with toxic or metabolic encephalopathies, including sepsis. They have the least association with seizures.

10. Occipital-predominant GRDA are common in children and may rarely be associated with a generalized epilepsy syndrome (e.g., childhood absence epilepsy).
11. LRDA is an epileptogenic pattern seen in critically ill patients with structural lesions; TIRDA is a subtype of LRDA associated with mesial temporal lobe epilepsy.
12. GPDs are a common pattern in critically ill patients associated with nonconvulsive seizures. Triphasic waves are a subtype of GPDs with triphasic morphology and usually an anterior–posterior or less commonly a posterior–anterior lag.
13. Triphasic waves may be potentially ictal or nonictal. These can be distinguished based on their electrographic features and response to a trial of antiepileptic medications.
14. LPDs are highly epileptogenic patterns and represent the electrographic markers of an acute destructive process of the underlying cortex.
15. Ictal LPDs can be identified based on their clinical accompaniments, regional increase in cerebral metabolism, and electrographic features.
16. BIPDs are bilateral PDs and are usually asymmetric. They are less common compared to LPDs and are usually seen in severe encephalopathy.
17. GSW discharges of more than 2.5 Hz are potentially ictal patterns.
18. Determining the ictal potential of a repetitive pattern is the key to its appropriate management.

References

1. Hirsch LJ, Fong MWK, Leitinger M, et al. American Clinical Neurophysiology Society's Standardized Critical Care EEG terminology: 2021 version. *Journal of Clinical Neurophysiology*. 2021 Jan;**38**(1):1–29.

2. Pohlmann-Eden B, Hoch DB, Cochius JI, Chiappa KH. Periodic lateralized epileptiform discharges – a critical review. *Journal of Clinical Neurophysiology*. 1996 Nov 1;**13**(6):519–30.

3. Chong DJ, Hirsch LJ. Which EEG patterns warrant treatment in the critically ill? Reviewing the evidence for treatment of periodic epileptiform discharges and related patterns. *Journal of Clinical Neurophysiology*. 2005 Apr 1;**22**(2):79–91.

4. Hirsch LJ, Claassen J, Mayer SA, Emerson RG. Stimulus-induced rhythmic, periodic, or ictal discharges (SIRPIDs): a common EEG phenomenon in the critically ill. *Epilepsia*. 2004 Feb;**45**(2):109–23.

5. Accolla EA, Kaplan PW, Maeder-Ingvar M, Jukopila S, Rossetti AO. Clinical correlates of frontal intermittent rhythmic delta activity (FIRDA). *Clinical Neurophysiology*. 2011 Jan 1;**122**(1):27–31.

6. Moeller F, Pressler RM, Cross JH. Genetic generalized epilepsy. In *Oxford Textbook of Clinical Neurophysiology* (p. 301). Oxford University Press, Oxford; 2016.

7. Gaspard N, Manganas L, Rampal N, Petroff OA, Hirsch LJ. Similarity of lateralized rhythmic delta activity to periodic lateralized epileptiform discharges in critically ill patients. *JAMA Neurology.* 2013 Oct 1;70(10):1288–95.

8. Di Gennaro G, Quarato PP, Onorati P, et al. Localizing significance of temporal intermittent rhythmic delta activity (TIRDA) in drug-resistant focal epilepsy. *Clinical Neurophysiology.* 2003 Jan 1;114(1):70–8.

9. Foreman B, Claassen J, Khaled KA, et al. Generalized periodic discharges in the critically ill: a case-control study of 200 patients. *Neurology.* 2012 Nov 6;**79** (19):1951–60.

10. Jadeja N, Zarnegar R, Legatt AD. Clinical outcomes in patients with generalized periodic discharges. *Seizure.* 2017 Feb 1;45:114–18.

11. O'Rourke D, Chen PM, Gaspard N, et al. Response rates to anticonvulsant trials in patients with triphasic-wave EEG patterns of uncertain significance. *Neurocritical Care.* 2016 Apr 1;24(2):233–9.

12. Boulanger JM, Deacon C, Lécuyer D, Gosselin S, Reiher J. Triphasic waves versus nonconvulsive status epilepticus: EEG distinction. *Canadian Journal of Neurological Sciences.* 2006 Jul;33(2):175–80.

13. Glauser T, Shinnar S, Gloss D, et al. Evidence-based guideline: treatment of convulsive status epilepticus in children and adults: report of the Guideline Committee of the American Epilepsy Society. *Epilepsy Currents.* 2016 Jan;**16** (1):48–61.

14. Punia V, Garcia CG, Hantus S. Incidence of recurrent seizures following hospital discharge in patients with LPDs (PLEDs) and nonconvulsive seizures recorded on continuous EEG in the critical care setting. *Epilepsy and Behavior.* 2015 Aug 1;49:250–54.

15. Ruiz AR, Vlachy J, Lee JW, et al. Association of periodic and rhythmic electro-encephalographic patterns with seizures in critically ill patients. *JAMA Neurology.* 2017 Feb 1;74(2):181–8.

16. Herman ST, Abend NS, Bleck TP, et al. Consensus statement on continuous EEG in critically ill adults and children, part I: indications. *Journal of Clinical Neurophysiology.* 2015 Apr;32(2):87.

17. Maciel CB, Gilmore EJ. Seizures and epileptiform patterns in SAH and their relation to outcomes. *Journal of Clinical Neurophysiology.* 2016 Jun 1;**33** (3):183–95.

18. Claassen J, Jette N, Chum F, et al. Electrographic seizures and periodic discharges after intracerebral hemorrhage. *Neurology.* 2007 Sep 25;**69**(13):1356–65.

19. Fitzpatrick W, Lowry N. PLEDs: clinical correlates. *Canadian Journal of Neurological Sciences*. 2007 Nov 1;**34**(4):443–50.

20. Struck AF, Westover MB, Hall LT, et al. Metabolic correlates of the ictal-interictal continuum: FDG-PET during continuous EEG. *Neurocritical Care*. 2016 Jun 1;**24**(3):324–31.

21. Li HT, Wu T, Lin WR, et al. Clinical correlation and prognostic implication of periodic EEG patterns: a cohort study. *Epilepsy Research*. 2017 Mar 1;**131**:44–50.

Chapter 16

Ictal Patterns (Electrographic Seizures)

Ictal patterns are repetitive abnormalities that electrographically represent ongoing seizure activity.

The identification of ictal patterns is largely based on their clinical accompaniments and electrographic features. Evidence of regional hypermetabolism (PET) or increased blood flow (SPECT) on nuclear imaging techniques may also suggest an ictal focus. The rationale for aggressive treatment of these patterns should be based on the possibility of clinical improvement with the resolution of the abnormality [1,2].

Clinically, ictal patterns may be accompanied by subtle focal manifestations such as clonic activity or altered mentation (nonconvulsive seizures).

Electrographically, the hallmark of an ictal pattern is "evolution." The presence of "plus features" also renders the pattern more ictal appearing than the same pattern without the plus feature (also known as a plus term) [3].

Evolution

An evolving pattern shows at least two sequential electrographic changes in frequency, morphology, or location. Changes in amplitude or sharpness alone do not qualify as evolution.

The individual change should persist for at least three cycles (three times) and not exceed 5 min in duration to qualify (e.g., a change is frequency as 3 Hz for 1 min to 2 Hz for 8 min to 1 Hz for 2 min doesn't qualify):

- At least two sequential frequency changes, which may be either increases (crescendo) or decreases (decrescendo) of more than 0.5 Hz each, will qualify.
- At least two sequential morphological changes to a new morphology will also qualify.
- Spreading in or out of at least two different electrode locations will also qualify.

If the pattern changes but doesn't meet the criteria for evolution, it is called a "fluctuating pattern." Static patterns refer to those that do not evolve or fluctuate [3]. Figure 16.1 shows an evolution in frequency, morphology, and spread.

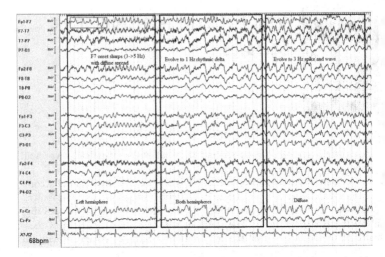

Figure 16.1 Seventy-seven-year-old with altered mentation, onset is characterized by low amplitude LPDs (3 Hz) in the Fp1 channel that initially evolves to diffuse low amplitude sharply contoured theta (5–6 Hz) [*frequency*] followed by frontal-predominant higher amplitude rhythmic delta (1 Hz) with embedded spikes [*morphology*] that spread to both hemispheres [*location*] and then increase in frequency to frontal-predominant generalized spike-wave discharges (2–3 Hz) before abruptly terminating (time base 15 s). Therefore, in this example, the original waveform evolves in frequency, morphology, and location (spread) constituting an electrographic seizure.

"Plus" Term

As discussed before, the presence of a "plus" feature also renders the repetitive pattern more ictal in appearance. LPD with plus features (usually superimposed low-amplitude fast activity or "F") are much more likely to be associated with epileptic seizures compared to those without plus features (as high as 74% based on a single study) [3,4].

Use the following "plus terms" with the combination of main terms as follows:

+ F: for superimposed low amplitude fast activity (e.g., GPD+F). See Figure 16.2.
+ R: for superimposed rhythmic delta activity (e.g., GPD+R). See Figure 16.3.
+ S: for superimposed sharp waves or spikes (e.g., Left LRDA+S). See Figure 16.4.

The term plus fast (+F) may be applied to both periodic discharges and rhythmic delta activity. Plus sharp (+S) is not applicable to periodic discharges

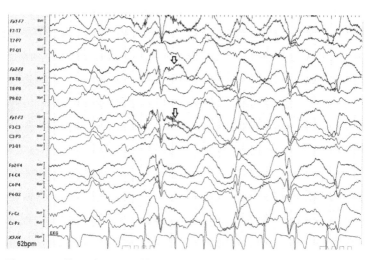

Figure 16.2 Thirty-three-year-old man with generalized epilepsy, GPDs with plus F features (fast). Brush-like low-amplitude rhythmic fast activity with a frontal predominance overrides the periodic discharge.

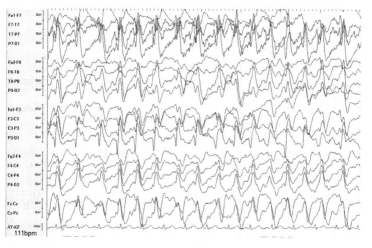

Figure 16.3 Same patient as in Figure 16.2, GPDs with plus R features (rhythmic) seen during a seizure. Spikes should not be time locked to slow waves, else they qualify as spike and wave (SW) instead of PD plus S.

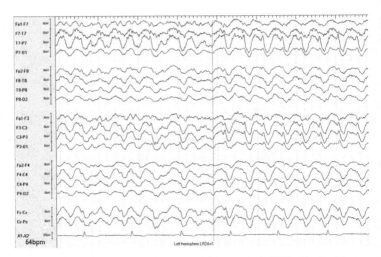

Figure 16.4 Same patient as in Figure 16.1, left hemispheric LRDA with plus S features (sharps). Low-amplitude sharps override the rhythmic waveforms.

as they are inherently sharp; conversely, plus rhythmic (+R) is not applicable to rhythmic delta activity as this is inherently rhythmic. Generally, plus features do not apply to spike and wave complexes.

Electrographic Seizures

Electrographic seizures (nonconvulsive or subclinical seizures) are epileptic seizures diagnosed on EEG alone. They occur without obvious clinical accompaniments.

Conventionally, an electrographic seizure has a clear start (onset) followed by evolution and termination (offset) with a duration that by convention is 10 s or more. Voltage attenuation (suppression) or slowing may be seen immediately postseizure. The seizure pattern may consist of evolving rhythmic activity (alpha, theta, or delta range), sharp/spike waves, fast activity (beta range), periods of attenuation, or combinations of these.

Heralding discharges (such as spikes) may occur immediately prior to onset and periodic discharges are common post offset (e.g., post ictal LPDs).

Electrocardiographic abnormalities such as tachycardia and less commonly bradycardia or asystole may be seen on the EKG channel during the seizure. In neonates and young children, ictal apneas may also occur.

Electrographic seizures are defined as patterns of 10 s or more in duration with on any one of three criteria (Salzburg criteria) [3,5,6]:

1. repetitive epileptic discharges of frequency greater than 2.5 Hz; OR,
2. repetitive epileptic discharges or rhythmic slowing of frequency less than 2.5 Hz AND shows at least one of the following features:

   a. clinical accompaniments (may be subtle); these are referred to as "electroclinical" seizures.
   b. spatiotemporal evolution as described above.
   c. significant clinical and EEG improvement after a trial of antiepileptic medication (EEG improvement as described before must not be limited to the suppression of discharges, but emergence of previously absent normal features such as a posterior dominant rhythm).

Figures 16.5 to 16.11 show the sequential progression of atypical electrographic seizure from onset to termination.

The reader should note that the "10 s" rule is an adopted convention. Electroclinical seizures (i.e., those with a definite clinical correlate time locked to an EEG pattern, such as face or limb twitching) are classified seizures even if the accompanying electrographic pattern may be less than 10 s.

Clinical Implications of Nonconvulsive Seizures

1. Seizures occur in 8%–20% of critically ill patients with altered mentation; they are almost always nonconvulsive. These patients may not have acute brain injury or prior epilepsy [7].
2. Nonconvulsive seizures (NCS) or nonconvulsive status epilepticus (NCSE) may lead to persistently abnormal mentation despite apparent successful treatment of convulsive status epilepticus (CSE). During 24 hours of continuous EEG monitoring after CSE, NCS was recorded in 48% and NCSE in 14% in one large study [8].
3. Continuous EEG monitoring is the preferred method of diagnosis for nonconvulsive seizures as there can be several hours of delay before the first seizure is recorded. Typical 30- to 60-min recordings identify NCS in only 45%–58% of patients in whom seizures are eventually recorded [9].
4. The duration of continuous EEG monitoring should be tailored to the individual patient. Recording for at least 24 hours is recommended, and this should be extended to at least 48–72 hours in high-risk patients (those who are comatose, have prior seizures, are pharmacologically sedated, are undergoing antiepileptic drug withdrawal, or have epileptogenic abnormalities such as periodic discharges on EEG). Noncomatose

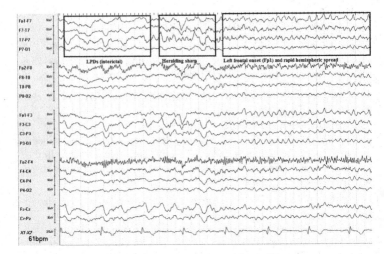

Figure 16.5 Same patient as in Figure 16.1; this electrographic seizure onset is characterized by a sharp theta activity (5–6 Hz) in the Fp1 channel followed by rapid left hemispheric spread. A heralding sharp wave at Fp1 precedes the onset.

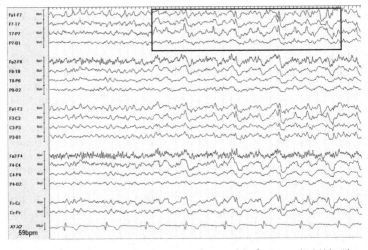

Figure 16.6 Sharp theta seen in Figure 16.5 slows to delta frequency (1–3 Hz) with emergence of embedded left hemispheric LPDs (1 Hz) with wide fields as the seizure continues.

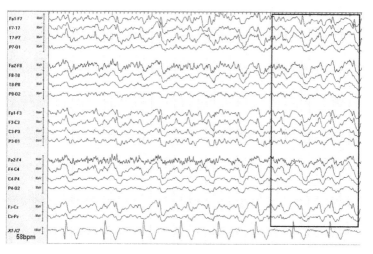

Figure 16.7 LPDs seen in Figure 16.6 become rhythmic and increase in frequency, transforming into 3 Hz LRDA (left hemisphere) with embedded sharps (LRDA plus S) as the seizure continues. This pattern has a wide bilateral field (secondary generalization).

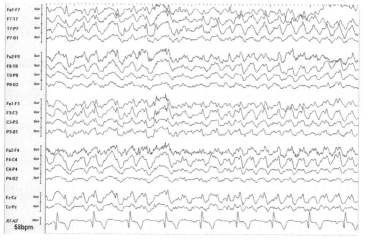

Figure 16.8 Approximately 3 Hz LRDA plus S seen in Figure 16.7 evolves in morphology to a lower amplitude and sharps become less prominent.

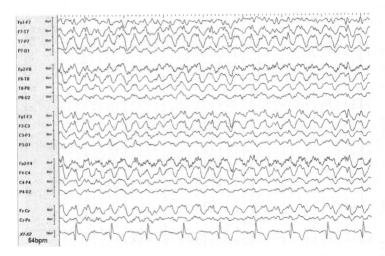

Figure 16.9 Lateralized rhythmic delta plus S seen in Figures 16.7 and 16.8 continues for about 7–8 s during the seizure.

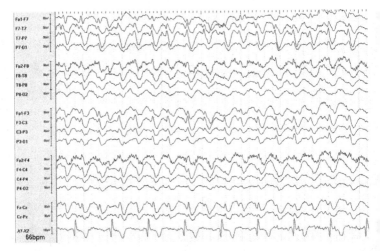

Figure 16.10 LRDA plus S seen in Figure 16.9 slightly decreases in frequency during this part of the seizure.

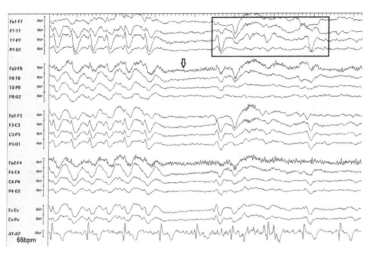

Figure 16.11 The seizure abruptly terminates, followed by a brief period of generalized suppression (postictal generalized suppression) and reemergence of left hemispheric LPDs (post ictal LPDs).

patients without prior seizures or early epileptogenic abnormalities (within 30–120 mins on EEG) have a very low risk of seizures (<5%) based on multiple studies [10,11].

5. Both NCS and NCSE are associated with increased mortality based on multiple studies, with the underlying etiology being the key prognostic factor [12,13].

6. Longer duration and greater delay in the diagnosis of NCS may contribute to worse outcomes. There is growing evidence to suggest that NCS may be associated with neuronal injury [14].

Brief Potentially Ictal Rhythmic Discharges (BIRDs)

These are typically focal sharply contoured bursts of less than 10 s duration that may show evolution or epileptic discharges. These are occasionally seen in critically ill adults with altered mentation and underlying structural injuries (e.g., strokes or tumors). Those with BIRDs are more likely to have seizures, and some may have only nonconvulsive seizures (epileptogenic). Their prognostic significance is not known [15]. Figure 16.12 shows an example of a BIRD.

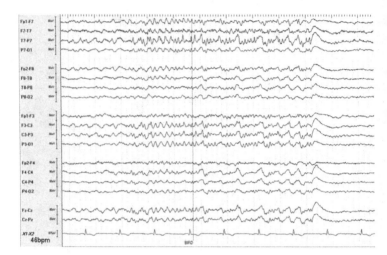

Figure 16.12 Same patient as in Figure 16.1, a brief potentially ictal rhythmic discharge (BIRD) seen during treatment of nonconvulsive status epilepticus (time base 10 s).

Chapter Summary

1. Ictal patterns represent ongoing electrographic seizures. They are recognized by their clinical accompaniments (may be subtle) and electrographic features.
2. Evolution is the electrographic hallmark of an ictal pattern, plus features (such as overriding fast activity) also render a pattern more ictal in appearance.
3. Electrographic seizures will typically have a clear onset, evolution, and offset. Conventionally, they should last for 10 s or more.
4. Electrographic seizures are common after convulsive seizures, in acute brain injury, and in critically ill patients with altered mentation.
5. Continuous EEG monitoring is the preferred method of diagnosing electrographic seizures. Typically, a duration of 24 hours is sufficient, but this should be extended in certain high-risk populations.

References

1. Cole AJ. Status epilepticus and periictal imaging. *Epilepsia*. 2004 Jul;**45**:72–77.

2. Jirsch J, Hirsch LJ. Nonconvulsive seizures: developing a rational approach to the diagnosis and management in the critically ill population. *Clinical Neurophysiology*. 2007 Aug;**118**(8):1660–70.

3. Hirsch LJ, Fong MWK, Leitinger M, et al. American Clinical Neurophysiology Society's Standardized Critical Care EEG terminology: 2021 version. *Journal of Clinical Neurophysiology.* 2021 Jan;**38**(1):1–29.

4. Reiher J, Rivest J, Maison FG, Leduc CP. Periodic lateralized epileptiform discharges with transitional rhythmic discharges: association with seizures. *Electroencephalography and Clinical Neurophysiology.* 1991 Jan 1;**78**(1):12–17.

5. Beniczky S, Hirsch LJ, Kaplan PW, et al. Unified EEG terminology and criteria for nonconvulsive status epilepticus. *Epilepsia.* 2013 Sep;**54**:28–29.

6. Leitinger M, Trinka E, Gardella E, et al. Diagnostic accuracy of the Salzburg EEG criteria for non-convulsive status epilepticus: a retrospective study. *The Lancet Neurology.* 2016 Sep 1;**15**(10):1054–62.

7. Laccheo I, Sonmezturk H, Bhatt AB, et al. Non-convulsive status epilepticus and non-convulsive seizures in neurological ICU patients. *Neurocritical Care.* 2015 Apr 1;**22**(2):202–11.

8. DeLorenzo RJ, Waterhouse EJ, Towne AR, et al. Persistent nonconvulsive status epilepticus after the control of convulsive status epilepticus. *Epilepsia.* 1998 Aug;**39**(8):833–40.

9. Claassen J, Mayer SA, Kowalski RG, Emerson RG, Hirsch LJ. Detection of electrographic seizures with continuous EEG monitoring in critically ill patients. *Neurology.* 2004 May 25;**62**(10):1743–48.

10. Herman ST, Abend NS, Bleck TP, et al. Consensus statement on continuous EEG in critically ill adults and children, part I: indications. *Journal of Clinical Neurophysiology.* 2015 Apr;**32**(2):87.

11. Struck AF, Osman G, Rampal N, et al. Time-dependent risk of seizures in critically ill patients on continuous electroencephalogram. *Annals of Neurology.* 2017 Aug;**82**(2):177–85.

12. De Marchis GM, Pugin D, Meyers E, et al. Seizure burden in subarachnoid hemorrhage associated with functional and cognitive outcome. *Neurology.* 2016 Jan 19;**86**(3):253–60.

13. Foreman B, Claassen J, Khaled KA, et al. Generalized periodic discharges in the critically ill: a case-control study of 200 patients. *Neurology.* 2012 Nov 6;**79**(19):1951–60.

14. Kaplan PW. Prognosis in nonconvulsive status epilepticus. In *Prognosis of epilepsies* (pp. 311–25). John Libbey Eurotext, Paris; 2003.

15. Yoo JY, Rampal N, Petroff OA, Hirsch LJ, Gaspard N. Brief potentially ictal rhythmic discharges in critically ill adults. *JAMA Neurology.* 2014 Apr 1;**71**(4):454–62.

Activation Procedures

Activation procedures are provocative maneuvers that can elicit epileptiform abnormalities in susceptible individuals. Two commonly employed activation procedures are hyperventilation and photic stimulation. Prior sleep deprivation may be used to increase the yield of an EEG but isn't considered a "maneuver."

Hyperventilation (HV)

Procedure

The patient is asked to take deep regular breaths at 20–30 times per minute for about 3–5 min (or sooner if they wish) and the EEG recording is continued for at least 3 min afterward. Balloons or toy windmills are helpful in children.

Contraindications

Cerebrovascular, cardiac, and pulmonary diseases, sickle cell disorder, and Moya-Moya disease are important contraindications.

Description

The effort, clinical effects (symptoms, seizures, or nonepileptic attacks) and the EEG response are noted. Sinus tachycardia is commonly seen in the single EKG channel; Hyperventilation must be stopped if ST segment changes or arrythmias are noted.

Normal Electrographic Response

A symmetric high-amplitude generalized background slowing with a frontal predominance is typical in children and young adults (called buildup). This response is age dependent and may be absent in older individuals. Figure 17.1 shows a prominent HV related build up in a child, Figure 17.2 shows a milder response in an adolescent.

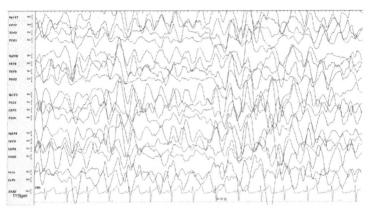

Figure 17.1 Five-year-old boy undergoing HV, symmetrical high-amplitude generalized delta slowing characteristic of a normal buildup.

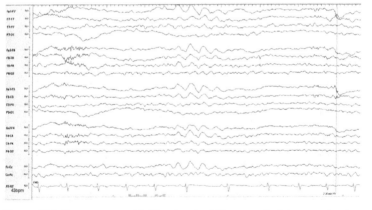

Figure 17.2 Seventeen-year-old girl undergoing HV, comparatively less prominent buildup.

Abnormal Responses

1. Seizures (commonly absences) or epileptic discharges may be elicited in certain generalized epilepsies such as childhood absence epilepsy (CAE). Figure 17.3 shows an absence seizure triggered after HV.

2. HV-induced build up should typically disappear as soon as normal breathing is resumed. Prolonged build up that persists beyond 1 min of stopping hyperventilation is nonspecific but may be associated hypoglycemia (resolves after a snack) or cerebrovascular disease such as Moya-Moya. Figure 17.4 shows prolonged hyperventilation build up associated with Moya-Moya disease.

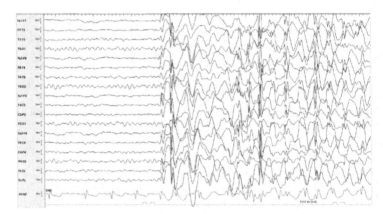

Figure 17.3 Twelve-year-old boy with CAE, absence seizure-induced post HV.

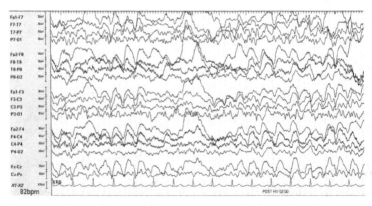

Figure 17.4 Nineteen-year-old woman with Moya-Moya disease, prolonged HV buildup.

3. Asymmetric response or focal slowing may be seen in older individuals with atherosclerotic cerebrovascular disease [1,2].

Photic Stimulation (PS)

Intermittent photic stimulation is best performed a few minutes after hyperventilation. This technique is useful in diagnosing photosensitive epilepsies and tailoring individual treatments.

Procedure

A series of 5 to 10 s blocks of photic stimulation are administered using a flashing lamp in a dimly lit room. At our institution, we start with a flash frequency of 1 Hz and increase in increments of 2 Hz to maximum of 30 Hz. The procedure should be stopped as soon as epileptiform discharges are seen to prevent provoking a seizure.

Contraindications

Photic stimulation is routinely performed as part of a standardized electroencephalogram. The risk of a provoked generalized tonic clonic seizure is very low (0.04%) [3].

Description

Any clinical effects such as myoclonus, absences, eyelid fluttering, and headaches should be recorded along with the flash frequency and EEG response. Nonepileptic attacks are also common.

Normal Electrographic Response

Symmetric photic driving response is characterized by repetitive sharp, positive waves that occur with an occipital dominance at the flash frequency or a slower harmonic. A fragmented or absent response is also normal. Figure 17.5 shows a normal photic driving response.

Abnormal Response

1. *Photo-Paroxysmal Response (PPR) consists of induction of epileptic discharges in response to photic stimulation.* The discharges may continue despite stopping the stimulation (self-sustaining response) or result in a seizure (photo convulsive response). Self-sustaining and self-limited responses have similar associations with epilepsy.
   Significance: Photo-paroxysmal responses are typically observed between 10 and 30 Hz. They are more common in young women. Eye closure during the stimulation enhances the response while drowsiness, non-REM sleep,

and medications such as Valproate may blunt it. Generalized responses are more common (e.g., JME, CAE, and JAE), but focal responses can also occur (idiopathic occipital epilepsy). Colors and patterns may also enhance the response. Figure 17.6 shows a generalized PPR (non-self-sustaining),

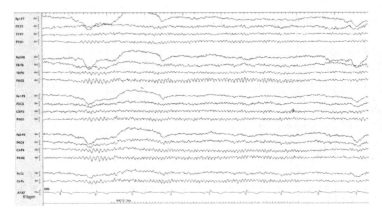

Figure 17.5 Thirty-two-year-old woman with migraines, normal driving response.

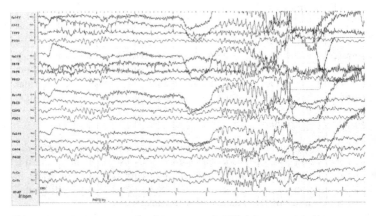

Figure 17.6 Twenty-seven-year-old woman with JME, photo-paroxysmal response at 9 Hz flash frequency characterized by frontally predominant rhythmic sharp discharges. Provoked discharges do not sustain beyond the photic stimulation.

Figure 17.7 shows a generalized PPR (self-sustaining), and Figure 17.8 shows a photo convulsive response.

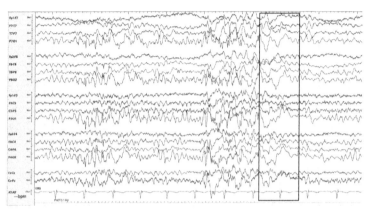

Figure 17.7 Eighteen-year-old woman with JME, photo-paroxysmal response at 11 Hz flash frequency characterized by occipital-predominant polyspikes wave discharges. Provoked discharges sustain beyond the photic stimulation.

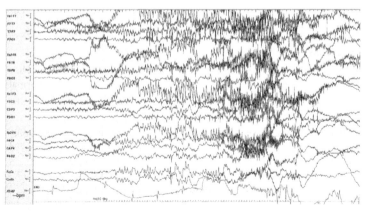

Figure 17.8 Same patient as in Figure 17.6, photo convulsive response at 15 Hz flash frequency. Note the generalized myogenic artifact (convulsion) that quickly obscures the discharges.

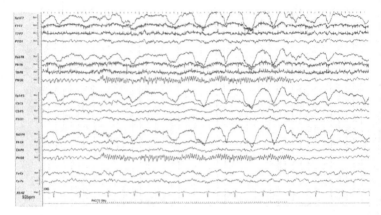

Figure 17.9 Twenty-three-year-old woman with migraines, asymmetric driving over the right occipital region.

2. An asymmetric driving response is not always abnormal, especially if present in isolation. It may suggest a structural focus on the absent side. The presence of a driving response in a blind individual may suggest psychogenic or cortical blindness. Figure 17.9 shows an asymmetric photic driving.

3. High-amplitude occipital spikes may be seen with progressive myoclonic epilepsies such as neuronal ceroid lipofuscinosis (NCL); these usually occur at lower flash frequencies (1 or 2 Hz) [3,4].

Artifactual Responses

These responses are the result of either physiological or external artifact. They have no pathological significance but may be confused with an abnormal response. These are commonly seen in the anterior channels (e.g., frontopolar).

1. Photo-myogenic (myoclonic) response occurs with prominent fast spiky muscle artifact in the representing facial muscle contractions time locked to the photic flash. Figure 17.10 shows photo myoclonic response.

2. Eye flutter artifact may also be seen with photic stimulation. Figure 17.9 shows eye flutter artifact in addition to asymmetric driving response.

3. Electrode artifact may occur in the frontal-polar channels, this may be synchronous with the photic flash (flash artifact).

4. Photic cell artifact (photovoltaic response) is like flash artifact but stops if the electrode is covered. Figure 17.11 shows a photocell artifact.

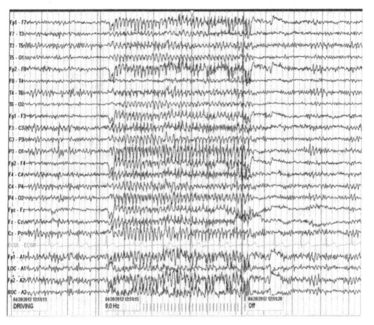

Figure 17.10 Photo myoclonic artifact at 8 Hz flash frequency.

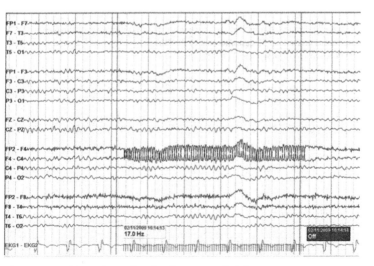

Figure 17.11 Photovoltaic cell artifact (F4) at 17 Hz flash frequency.

Chapter Summary

1. Activation procedures are used to elicit epileptic activity. Hyperventilation and photic stimulation are commonly used activation procedures.
2. Hyperventilation is contraindicated in cerebrovascular disease.
3. The normal hyperventilation response consists of a high-amplitude, frontally dominant, generalized slowing (called buildup). This is age dependent and may be absent in older patients.
4. Hyperventilation provokes absence seizures in childhood absence epilepsy (CAE). Prolonged buildup may be seen in Moya-Moya disease.
5. Photic stimulation normally results in symmetric, occipital-dominant, repetitive sharps at the flash frequency or a slower harmonic (called driving).
6. Abnormal photic responses include the photo-paroxysmal response which consists of induction of epileptic discharges with photic stimulation and the photo convulsive response results from a seizure elicited during photic stimulation.

References

1. Kane N, Grocott L, Kandler R, Lawrence S, Pang C. Hyperventilation during electroencephalography: safety and efficacy. *Seizure*. 2014 Feb 1;**23**(2):129–34.

2. Sunder TR, Erwin CW, Dubois PJ. Hyperventilation induced abnormalities in the electroencephalogram of children with moyamoya disease. *Electroencephalography and Clinical Neurophysiology*. 1980 Aug 1;**49**(3–4):414–20.

3. Kasteleijn-Nolst Trenité D, Rubboli G, Hirsch E, et al. Methodology of photic stimulation revisited: updated European algorithm for visual stimulation in the EEG laboratory. *Epilepsia*. 2012 Jan;**53**(1):16–24.

4. Elleder M, Franc J, Kraus J, et al. Neuronal ceroid lipofuscinosis in the Czech Republic: analysis of 57 cases. Report of the "Prague NCL group." *European Journal of Paediatric Neurology*. 1997 Jan 1;**1**(4):109–14.

Chapter

18

Common Seizure Mimics

Everything that shakes isn't a seizure. Before you determine the patient has experienced epileptic seizures, make sure to have considered relevant seizure mimics. These nonepileptic conditions imitate epileptic seizures and recurrences may be misdiagnosed as epilepsy.

A careful history, physical examination, and video EEG evaluation are useful in diagnosing the cause of paroxysmal "seizure-like" events. Less commonly, both epileptic and nonepileptic events may coexist, necessitating inquiry into whether the event in question is consistent with the patient's typical event and if other uncharacterized events also exist. A complete evaluation should aim to capture and characterize each of the patient's event type, though frequent events are easier to characterize than those occurring seldomly.

In a majority of conditions that imitate epileptic seizures, the EEG remains unchanged during the event. However, some nonepileptic conditions are associated with abnormal EEG patterns that should not be mistaken for ictal activity. This chapter lists common seizure mimics and their associated electrographic features.

Seizure mimics are grouped as physiological (organic disease) or psychological. Furthermore, physiological mimics may be neurologic, systemic, or both (such as syncope) [1].

Seizure Mimics

Neurological Mimics

- syncope
- transient ischemic attack (TIA)
- migraines
- parasomnias
- movement disorders

Systemic Mimics

- cardiac arrythmias
- transient toxicities and metabolic disturbances (such as hypoglycemia)

Psychological Mimics

- nonepileptic seizures and other conversion disorders
- panic attacks
- other behavioral, psychiatric, and psychological conditions

Neurological Seizure Mimics

Syncope

Syncope is characterized by a transient loss of consciousness and postural tone due to transitory global cerebral hypoperfusion. Often, there is accompanying brief multifocal tonic activity, eye deviation, vocalizations, hallucinations, and sphincteric disturbances (convulsive syncope) that can be mistaken for an epileptic seizure. Semiologically, syncopal events are brief, positional, and lack postictal confusion unlike epileptic seizures. Incontinence and lateral tongue bites are rare. Neurogenic (autonomic) and cardiogenic causes exist with vasovagal syncope being the most common cause.

The EEG during a syncope is characterized by emergence of generalized theta-delta slowing followed by a period of diffuse attenuation corresponding with transient cerebral hypoperfusion and resultant loss of consciousness. Recovery is characterized by the reemergence of generalized slowing followed by a return of the resting background. The EKG channel shows transient bradycardia or asystole [2]. Figures 18.1 to 18.4 show the sequence of EEG changes with syncope.

Rarely, epileptic seizures induce ictal or postictal cardiac arrythmias resulting in loss of consciousness [3]. Figure 18.5 shows EEG in postictal cardiac arrest.

Transient Ischemic Attacks (TIA)

Cerebrovascular accidents such as TIAs and strokes, unlike epileptic seizures are typically associated with negative symptoms (e.g., paralysis), though occasionally positive symptoms such as limb shaking occur, especially in the setting of bilateral carotid stenosis (limb shaking TIA) which may be mistaken for an epileptic seizure. The EEG is characterized by acute onset of focal slowing corresponding to the region of cerebral ischemia [4].

Migraines

Migraines with aura can mimic epileptic seizures. Migraine and epilepsy commonly coexist further complicating the diagnosis of individual events. Migraine

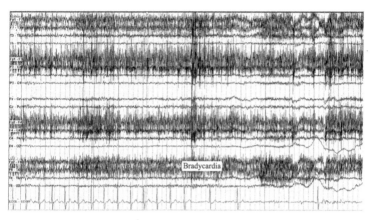

Figure 18.1 Fifty-three-year-old woman with convulsive syncope, sudden onset of bradycardia on EKG channel heralds the syncopal attack.

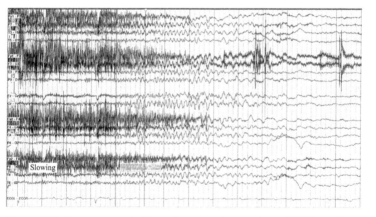

Figure 18.2 Same patient as in Figure 18.1, severe bradycardia on EKG followed by diffuse higher amplitude theta and delta slowing followed by attenuation.

may be associated with transient visual phenomena, focal motor, language, and sensory deficits and rarely in confusion, and coma. Sensory illusions and perceptional changes with hearing or vision (such as dramatic shrinking of body parts as a feature of "Alice in wonderland" syndrome) may also occur.

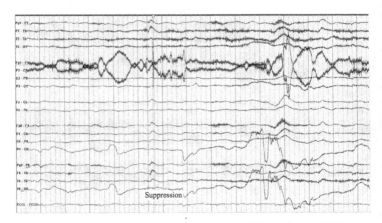

Figure 18.3 Same patient as in Figure 18.1, generalized EEG suppression (GES) with cardiac asystole.

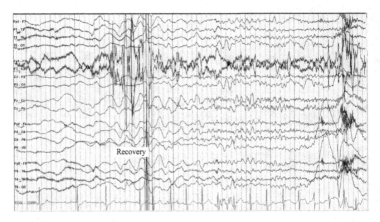

Figure 18.4 Same patient as in Figure 18.1, resolution of syncope characterized by diffuse slowing followed by rapid restoration of EEG background.

The EEG during migraines is usually normal but may show slowing (focal or diffuse) or amplitude attenuation (Figure 18.6). Though nonspecific, migraineurs have a higher incidence of photic driving [5,6].

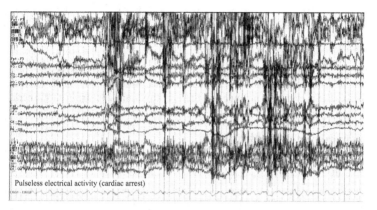

Pulseless electrical activity (cardiac arrest)

Figure 18.5 Fifty-year-old woman with postictal asystole, GES with pulseless electrical activity on EKG.

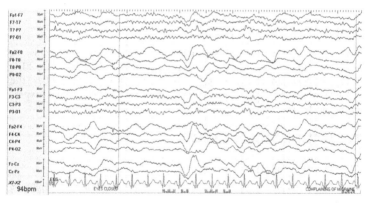

Figure 18.6 Thirty-year-old man with hemiplegic migraine, right hemisphere–predominant polymorphic delta slowing. Additionally, there is bilateral EKG artifact.

Parasomnias

Episodic sleep disorders (parasomnias) mimic nocturnal seizures. Epileptic seizures rarely occur during rapid eye movement (REM) sleep while parasomnias are specific to either REM or non-REM (slow-wave) sleep. The EEG can identify ictal activity and the sleep stage associated with the event. Sleep talking (somniloquy), sleep talking (somnambulism), confusional arousals, and night terrors occur during slow-wave sleep while REM behavior disorder and nightmares occur during REM sleep [7].

Movement Disorders

Movement disorders including tics, tremor, paroxysmal dyskinesias, and nonepileptic myoclonus are common seizure mimics. The EEG activity during these events is normal but there is rhythmic appearing movement artifact [7].

Systemic Seizure Mimics

Cardiac Arrythmias

Arrythmias related cardiogenic syncope are important to recognize as they may be life threatening. In long QT syndromes ventricular tachy-cardias may be triggered by emotions or exercise. Syncope in sleep, sensorineural deafness, and a family history of sudden death or drowning are important clues to this disorder. EKG channel may show abnormalities in heart rhythm [8].

Transient Toxicities or Metabolic Disturbances

Toxic and metabolic disturbances that lead to delirium, myoclonus, or transient deficits may mimic or precipitate seizure activity. The EEG usually shows nonspecific encephalopathy (Chapter 23 describes the EEG in encephalopathy). Hypoglycemia in particular, accentuates hyper-ventilation build up [8,9].

Psychological Seizure Mimics

Nonepileptic Seizures

Nonepileptic seizures (previously termed psychogenic seizures, nonepileptic attacks, or psuedoseizures) are behavioral events that resemble epileptic seizures without an electrographic correlate or clinical evidence of epilepsy. There may be a history of psychiatric comorbidities, emotional, or physical trauma. They commonly manifest with seizure-like movements and impaired consciousness, but unlike epileptic seizures, these typically have prominent proximal limb and truncal movements, side-to-side head movements, crying, and eye closure with resistance to passive opening. Epileptic seizures coexist in at least 10% of patients with nonepileptic seizures [10]. The EEG during the event shows a normal waking background (despite impaired consciousness) which may be obscured by movement artifact [11].

Panic Attacks

Panic (anxiety) attacks are episodes of fear, apprehension, or terror accompanied by hyperventilation, palpitations, chest pain, feeling faint or dizzy, paresthesia (around the mouth and fingers), and a feeling of chocking that lasts several minutes. The EEG is typically normal or shows hyperventilation build up. Rarely, insular seizures may resemble panic attacks.

Other Behavioral, Psychiatric, and Psychological Conditions

Many common pediatric behavioral conditions such as day dreaming, inattention, self-gratification (masturbation), eidetic imagery (vivid imaginations), temper tantrums, and out of body experiences mimic seizures. In adults, dissociative states, hallucinations, and occasionally fabricated or fictitious illness may mimic seizures. The EEG is normal during these events [8,12].

Chapter Summary

1. Think of seizure mimics before you diagnose epileptic seizures.
2. Some mimics, such as syncope, transient ischemic attacks (TIA), and migraines, may be associated with EEG abnormalities.
3. Seizure mimics may be neurological, systemic, or psychological.
4. Always confirm if the event in question is consistent with the patient's typical event, as the patient may have more than one type of event.
5. Though uncommon, both epileptic and nonepileptic events may coexist, hence it is important to characterize each of the patient's event types on video EEG.

References

1. Hopp JL. Nonepileptic episodic events. *CONTINUUM: Lifelong Learning in Neurology*. 2019 Apr 1;**25**(2):492–507.

2. Abubakr A, Wambacq I. The diagnostic value of EEGs in patients with syncope. *Epilepsy and Behavior*. 2005 May 1;**6**(3):433–4.

3. Duplyakov D, Golovina G, Lyukshina N, et al. Syncope, seizure-induced bradycardia and asystole: two cases and review of clinical and pathophysiological features. *Seizure*. 2014 Aug 1;**23**(7):506–11.

4. Bearden S, Uthman B. Cerebral hemodynamic compromise associated with limb shaking TIA and focal EEG slowing. *American Journal of Electroneurodiagnostic Technology*. 2009 Sep 1;**49**(3):225–43.

5. Smyth VO, Winter AL. The EEG in migraine. *Electroencephalography and Clinical Neurophysiology*. 1964 Jan 1;**16**(1–2):194–202.

6. Puca FM, De Tommaso M, Tota P, Sciruicchio V. Photic driving in migraine: correlations with clinical features. *Cephalalgia*. 1996 Jun;**16**(4):246–50.

7. Webb J, Long B, Koyfman A. An emergency medicine–focused review of seizure mimics. *Journal of Emergency Medicine.* 2017 May 1;**52**(5):645–53.

8. Brodtkorb E. Common imitators of epilepsy. *Acta Neurologica Scandinavica.* 2013 Jan;**127**:5–10.

9. Snogdal LS, Folkestad L, Elsborg R, et al. Detection of hypoglycemia associated EEG changes during sleep in type 1 diabetes mellitus. *Diabetes Research and Clinical Practice.* 2012 Oct 1;**98**(1):91–7.

10. Benbadis SR, Agrawal V, Tatum WO. How many patients with psychogenic nonepileptic seizures also have epilepsy? *Neurology.* 2001 Sep 11;**57**(5):915–17.

11. Syed TU, LaFrance WC Jr, Kahriman ES, et al. Can semiology predict psychogenic nonepileptic seizures? A prospective study. *Annals of Neurology.* 2011 Jun;**69**(6):997–1004.

12. Paolicchi JM. The spectrum of nonepileptic events in children. *Epilepsia.* 2002 Mar;**43**:60–4.

Chapter 19

Seizures

Seizures (epileptic seizures) are defined as transient symptomatic manifestations of abnormal excessive or synchronized neuronal activity of the brain.

They may be provoked due to acute cerebral insults (such as delirium, trauma or stroke), reflex (triggered by specific stimuli such as light or music), or unprovoked (epilepsy).

The International League Against Epilepsy (ILAE) has published a universal classification for seizures based primarily on consistent clinical observation of the seizure (semiology) and findings on ancillary tests such as the EEG and neuroimaging.

The ILAE classification (2017) distinguishes seizures into one of three types:

1. *Focal onset seizures* (previously: partial seizures) which originate within networks related to one hemisphere whether discrete or widely distributed within that hemisphere.
2. *Generalized onset seizures* (previously generalized seizures) which originate within and rapidly engage bilateral distributed networks.
3. *Unknown onset seizures* where the onset is not yet defined and a classification is not possible either due to a lack of observation of the onset or absence of a diagnostic evaluation (intended as a temporary category).

A 26-year-old woman reports brief episodes of déjà vu, rising abdominal feelings followed by confusion with lip smacking and right-hand fumbling. She has a history of febrile seizures as a child. Her brain MRI shows right mesial temporal sclerosis (MTS). A resting EEG shows sporadic right anterior temporal discharges and there is focal rhythmic activity originating over the right temporal channels during her episodes. Based on these focal features on seizure semiology (cognitive and autonomic aura at onset), neuroimaging (right MTS), and EEG (right temporal abnormalities), it may be inferred that her seizures originate within networks in the right hemisphere (mesial temporal lobe) – focal onset seizures.

On the other hand, A 17-year-old boy reports jerking and clumsiness in the morning, generalized convulsions precipitated by disco lights and binge drinking. He has a family history of epilepsy. His brain MRI is normal and resting EEG shows generalized spike and wave discharges. An ictal EEG has not been obtained. Based on generalized features in his semiology (myoclonus and convulsions) and interictal EEG as well as the absence of a focal abnormality on neuroimaging, it may be inferred that his seizures either originate or rapidly engage within both hemispheres – generalized onset seizures.

Classification of seizures into focal or generalized onset is a crucial first step toward understanding the patient's epilepsy (disorder of recurrent seizures). The diagnosis of epilepsy is described in Chapter 20. Further classification of seizures is optional but may be done based on two important observations of semiology:

1. impairment in awareness at any time during the seizure
2. observation of movements or motor activity at the very onset of the seizure

The remainder of this chapter discusses the application of these observations [1].

Focal Seizures

Focal (onset) seizures are categorized based on impairment of awareness (anytime during event), motor manifestations (at the very onset), and bilateral progression.

Impaired Awareness

1. *Focal seizures without impaired awareness (focal aware seizures):* The patient is fully aware of themselves and their surroundings throughout the seizure even if immobilized. They were previously called "simple" partial seizures. Motor, sensory, autonomic, or psychic symptoms with preservation of awareness and consciousness (aura) are common forms. Some progress to impairment of awareness or spread bilaterally (secondary generalization). A majority of this seizure type do not have an associated surface EEG correlate (70%–90%) though focal abnormalities (interictal sharps or slowing) or ictal rhythmic activity may occur [2].
2. *Focal seizures with impaired awareness (focal impaired awareness seizure):* If the patient's awareness becomes impaired (not necessarily unconscious) at any point during the seizure it is called a focal seizure with impaired awareness. They were previously called "complex" partial seizures or dyscognitive seizures. Typically, they last about 30 s to 3 min and are accompanied by purposeless movements (automatisms), amnesia, and other features such as aphasia depending on the region of cortical involvement. Some progress to secondary generalization. The EEG almost always shows focal abnormalities (interictal sharps/slowing) or ictal rhythmic activity with bilateral spread [1,2].

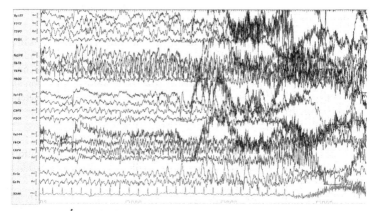

Figure 19.1 Twenty-three-year-old woman with temporal lobe epilepsy, focal onset (right hemisphere) evolves to bilateral tonic clonic (time base 20 s).

Motor Onset

1. *Focal seizures with motor onset (motor):* If the seizure onset is characterized by motor movements (due to increase or decrease in muscle contraction) then it is called a motor onset seizure. Any motor activity after onset of the seizure does not qualify as a motor seizure. Common forms of motor activity include automatisms, tonic or clonic activity, myoclonus, hyperkinetic movements, atonic activity, and epileptic spasms. The EEG shows myogenic or movement artifact along with ictal activity.
2. *Focal seizures with nonmotor onset (nonmotor):* If the seizure onset is not motor such as sensory, cognitive (aphasia), emotional, autonomic symptoms (aura), or behavioral arrest, then it is called a nonmotor seizure. The EEG may be normal or show ictal activity.

Focal to Bilateral Tonic Clonic

A focal onset seizure can spread bilaterally to become a bilateral tonic clonic seizure accompanied by loss of consciousness and convulsive activity (secondary generalization). The EEG shows spread of ictal activity into the contralateral hemisphere. Later parts of the record may be obscured by myogenic artifact [1]. Figure 19.1 shows bilateral tonic clonic evolution of a focal seizure.

Generalized Seizures

Generalized onset usually results in impaired awareness therefore these seizures are further classified based only on motor onset; not impairment of awareness.

1. *Generalized seizures with motor onset (motor):* The seizure onset is characterized by generalized (often symmetric) motor activity:

   - *Tonic clonic (GTCs) seizures* involve loss of consciousness and tonic extension of limbs (usually less than a minute) followed by rhythmic clonic jerking of the extremities. There may be associated apnea, incontinence, and tongue biting followed by prolonged postictal confusion or stupor. EEG shows generalized ictal activity that may be completely obscured by myogenic artifact. Figure 19.2 shows the tonic phase of a GTC while Figure 19.3 shows its clonic phase.
   - *Tonic seizures* involve sudden stiffening and arm extension for a few seconds. They may lead to falls and injury. EEG shows brief attenuation and/or burst of high-frequency fast activity with myogenic artifact (tonic) as shown in Figure 19.4.
   - *Atonic seizures* involve abrupt momentary loss of tone associated with head drop, falls, and injuries. EEG shows brief attenuation and/or slow spike wave discharges without myogenic artifact (atonic) as shown in Figure 19.5.
   - *Myoclonic seizures* involve sudden brief (milliseconds) bilateral jerks (esp. arms) that occur in clusters that may be triggered by photic or sensory stimulation. EEG shows generalized polyspikes/wave discharges with intermittent myogenic artifact (myogenic).
   - *Myoclonic-atonic seizures* involve myoclonic seizures (often multiple) followed by an atonic seizure, that may result in a drop attack. EEG shows a generalized discharge (myoclonic component) followed by after going high-voltage slow wave (atonic component).

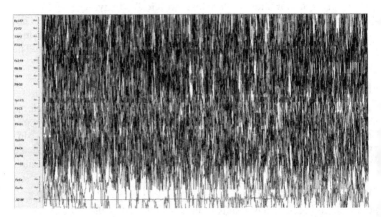

Figure 19.2 Same patient as in Figure 19.1, tonic phase of the GTC showing continuous myogenic artifact obscuring the recording.

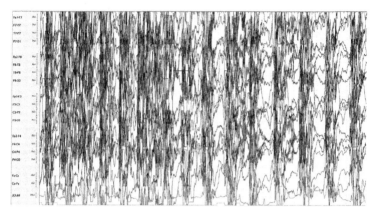

Figure 19.3 Same patient as in Figure 19.1, clonic phase of GTC showing periodic myogenic artifact obscuring the recording.

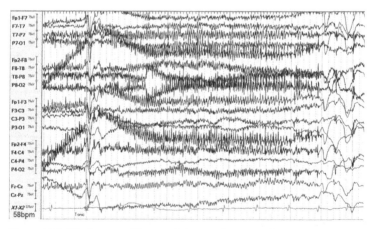

Figure 19.4 Fifty-four-year-old man with Lennox–Gastaut syndrome, tonic seizure characterized by brief generalized attenuation and low-voltage fast activity with overlying myogenic artifact.

- *Epileptic spams* involve sudden brief (1–2 s) extensor, flexor, or mixed posturing of the proximal limbs or trunk in quick series. They may be subtle such as chin movements, head nodding, or grimacing. EEG abnormalities are enhanced with sleep or arousal and consist of high-voltage sharps/slow

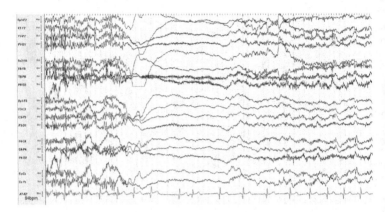

Figure 19.5 Same patient as in Figure 19.4, atonic seizure characterized by brief attenuation with slow spike and wave discharges. Note the absence of myogenic artifact.

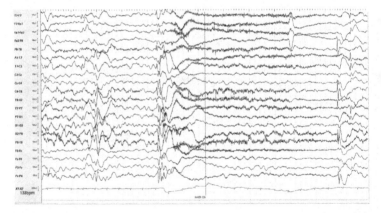

Figure 19.6 Nine-month-old boy with West syndrome, epileptic spasms characterized by high-voltage sharps/slow wave followed by low-amplitude fast activity and voltage attenuation (sensitivity of 20 uV).

wave followed by low-amplitude fast activity and voltage attenuation as shown in Figure 19.6. It may be generalized (for generalized onset spasms) or focal (for focal onset spasms). These ictal patterns may occur multiple times in sleep without the accompanying clinical spasm.

2. *Generalized seizures with nonmotor onset (nonmotor):* The seizure onset is characterized by the absence of motor movements, though some motor phenomena such as myoclonus or automatisms may follow. They were previously called absence seizures.

- *Typical absences* are characterized by abrupt onset and offset of impaired awareness usually associated with clonic movements of facial/perioral muscles. Absence status epilepticus may also occur. EEG shows regular 3 Hz generalized spike and wave discharges (GSW) in childhood absence epilepsy, faster irregular 3.5–6 Hz GSW and polyspikes and wave discharges may occur with later onsets. Figure 19.7 shows typical absences.

- *Atypical absences* are characterized by less abrupt onsets/offsets often associated with gradual head, truncal, or limb slumping and subtle myoclonus with only slight impairment in awareness. These are often seen in the intellectually impaired. EEG shows ongoing slow (less than 2.5 Hz) generalized spike and wave which is accentuated by hyperventilation. Figure 19.8 shows atypical absences.

- *Myoclonic absences* are characterized by rhythmic jerking of the arms, shoulders, and tonic abduction (arms lift up) with impaired awareness. EEG shows regular 3 Hz GSW with associated myoclonic artifact.

- *Absences with eyelid myoclonia* are characterized by brief, repetitive eye lid jerking with upward deviation of eyeballs and head extension. EEG shows high-amplitude generalized spike and wave/polyspikes and wave discharges at 3–6 Hz, provoked by photic stimulation. Figure 19.9 shows absences with eyelid myoclonia during photic stimulation.

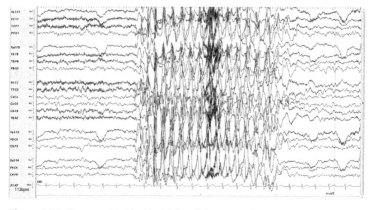

Figure 19.7 Ten-year-old girl with childhood absence epilepsy, typical absences showing a 3 Hz GSW discharges.

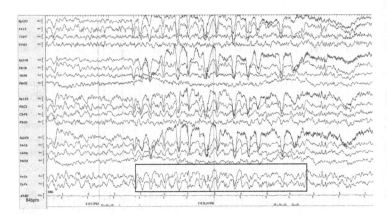

Figure 19.8 Same patient as in Figure 19.4, atypical absences with slow (2 Hz) generalized spike and wave discharges.

Neonatal Seizures

Seizures in neonates have focal onsets and are secondary to acute illness. They may be purely electrographic (particularly, in the critically ill) or associated with motor (such as automatisms, myoclonus, or spasms) or nonmotor onsets (autonomic or behavior arrest). For these reasons, neonatal seizures may not fit into the ILAE classification for older children and adults. The same clinical seizure type may at times, occur with or without electrographic correlate (electroclinical dissociation). Electrographically neonatal seizures are characterized by sudden, repetitive evolving stereotypical patterns with a definite onset and end but this definition has not been standardized. Their duration may be shorter than 10 s (such as BIRDs) [3]. Figure 19.10 shows a neonatal seizure.

The classification of seizure onset based on consistent clinical observation (focal or generalized onset), EEG and imaging findings forms the basis for diagnosing an epilepsy disorder as outlined in the following chapter (Chapter 20). Unknown onset seizures may also be classified as motor or nonmotor until their onset can be determined [1,4].

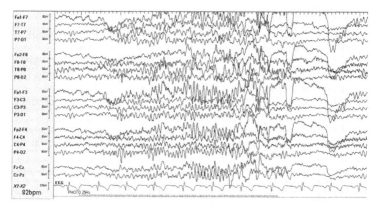

Figure 19.9 Eighteen-year-old woman with Jeavons syndrome, absences with eyelid myoclonia triggered by photic stimulation.

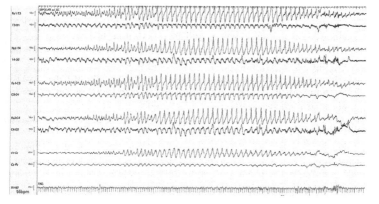

Figure 19.10 One-day-old boy with hypoxic ischemic encephalopathy, neonatal seizures characterized by evolving rhythmic activity (sensitivity 30 uV, time base 2 min).

Chapter Summary

1. Seizures (epileptic) are manifestations of transient abnormal excessive or synchronized cerebral neuronal activity.
2. Seizures may be provoked (acute conditions) or unprovoked (epilepsy).
3. Seizures are classified as focal or generalized onset based on consistent clinical observation, EEG, and imaging findings.
4. Focal onset seizures originate from a single hemisphere, while generalized seizures originate from bilateral hemispheres.
5. Focal seizures may be further classified based on impairment of awareness (anytime during seizure) and motor or nonmotor activity (at the very onset).
6. Focal seizures without impaired awareness may not have surface EEG abnormalities.
7. Focal seizures may secondarily generalize; these are now called focal to bilateral tonic clonic seizures.
8. Generalized seizures are associated with impaired awareness, hence only motor or nonmotor activity at onset is used to classify them.
9. Common generalized motor seizures include generalized tonic clonic seizures (GTCs), tonic, atonic, myoclonic, myoclonic-atonic, and epileptic spasms.
10. Common generalized nonmotor seizures include typical and atypical absences, myoclonic absences, and absences with eyelid myoclonia.
11. Additional features of the seizure occurring after onset that may be relevant to its propagation can be added as descriptors.
12. If the onset of a seizure is yet undefined, it may be temporarily referred to as an unknown onset seizure until a further determination can be made about its probable onset.

References

1. Fisher RS, Cross JH, French JA, et al. Operational classification of seizure types by the International League against Epilepsy: position paper of the ILAE Commission for Classification and Terminology. *Epilepsia*. 2017 Apr;58(4):522–30.

2. Verma A, Radtke R. EEG of partial seizures. *Journal of Clinical Neurophysiology*. 2006 Aug 1;23(4):333–9.

3. Pressler RM, Cilio MR, Mizrahi EM, et al. The ILAE classification of seizures and the epilepsies: modification for seizures in the neonate. Proposal from the ILAE Task Force on Neonatal Seizures.

4. Berg AT, Berkovic SF, Brodie MJ, et al. Revised terminology and concepts for organization of seizures and epilepsies: report of the ILAE Commission on Classification and Terminology, 2005–2009. *Epilepsia*. 2010 Apr;51(4):676–85.

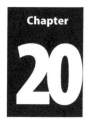

Chapter 20

Epilepsies

Making a Diagnosis of Epilepsy

Epilepsy is a disorder of recurrent unprovoked (or reflex) seizures. The key to the diagnosis of epilepsy is estimating the risk of seizure recurrence.

It may be diagnosed if at least two unprovoked (or reflex) seizures occur at least 24 hours apart. Studies have established that the risk of seizure recurrence after two unprovoked seizures is greater than 50% over the next 10 years, it is even higher after three unprovoked seizures.

However, epilepsy may also be diagnosed after a first-time seizure if the clinician estimates that the risk of future recurrences is high (similar to that after at least two seizures) or if there is evidence of an underlying epilepsy syndrome [1].

A history of prior brain insult, epileptogenic abnormalities on EEG, significant brain imaging abnormalities or nocturnal seizures confer an increased risk of future recurrence after a first-time seizure; enabling a diagnosis of epilepsy in the appropriate clinical context [2].

Conversely, epilepsy may be considered "resolved" for those who have outgrown an age-dependent epilepsy syndrome (Chapter 21 describes epilepsy syndromes) and those who have been seizure-free for at least 10 years with the last 5 years off antiseizure medications [1,2].

Describing the Epilepsy Disorder

Once you have diagnosed a patient with epilepsy, the next step is to classify it. The following approach is based on the ILAE classification of epilepsies [3]:

1. The first step is to diagnose the prevalent seizure type(s) as described in Chapter 19.
2. Next, diagnose the type of epilepsy based on the prevalent seizure type(s), comorbidities, and ancillary findings such as EEG (interictal and ictal) and neuroimaging abnormalities.
3. Focal onset seizures suggest focal epilepsy, generalized onset seizures suggest a generalized epilepsy and the presence of both seizure types suggests a mixed epilepsy.

4. Once you have determined the type of epilepsy (focal, generalized, or mixed), then consider if it fits into an epilepsy syndrome (often age specific). Focal epilepsies may or may not be syndromic, while generalized epilepsies are usually syndromic. Epilepsy syndromes are discussed in Chapter 21.

5. Finally, whether or not the epilepsy is syndromic, it is important to consider potential underlying etiologies.

6. Etiologically, epilepsies may be due to a structural (e.g., stroke) or genetic (e.g., SCN1A mutation with Dravet syndrome), infectious (e.g., neurocysticercosis), immune (e.g., anti-NMDA receptor encephalitis), or metabolic causes (e.g., pyridoxine dependent seizures). Not infrequently, the etiology is unknown.

With these steps, you will be able to comprehensively describe the epilepsy disorder.

Types of Epilepsies

Focal Epilepsy

Focal epilepsies are characterized by focal onset seizures types. Focal interictal and ictal EEG abnormalities (slowing or discharges) and neuroimaging findings (lesions) are supportive. Some focal epilepsies are syndromic. Focal epilepsies are subclassified as unifocal, hemispheric, or multifocal, they may also be grouped based on lobar involvement.

Frontal Lobe Epilepsy: Frontal lobe epilepsy is typically characterized by motor seizures (hyperkinetic or asymmetric tonic posturing), awareness may or may not be impaired. These seizures are typically nocturnal (arising out of non–rapid eye movement sleep) and often cluster. The interictal EEG is often normal though repeated EEGs may show epileptogenic discharges which may appear bifrontal or midline. The ictal EEG is often difficult to interpret, it may be normal or completely obscured by movement artifact during the seizure. Less commonly, a focal frontal ictal pattern may occur. Ictal patterns may be preceded by focal or diffuse suppression and/or low-voltage fast activity. False localization of the ictal pattern to the ipsilateral temporal lobe or false generalization (secondary bilateral synchronization) may also occur [4]. Figure 20.1 shows a frontal lobe seizure.

Temporal Lobe Epilepsy: Temporal lobe epilepsy is typically characterized by focal onset impaired awareness and nonmotor seizures (behavioral arrest). Temporal seizures may originate from the mesial or lateral parts of the temporal lobe as described:

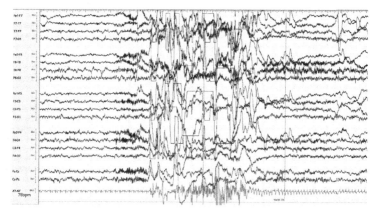

Figure 20.1 Seventeen-year-old girl with frontal lobe epilepsy, frontal-predominant high-amplitude discharges (midline channels), and movement artifact during nocturnal seizure (time base 60 s).

1. Mesial temporal lobe epilepsy typically has autonomic (rising epigastric sensation/abdominal discomfort), sensory (olfactory/gustatory), cognitive (déjà vu/jamais vu), or emotional (fear) onset seizures. Impaired awareness, behavioral arrest, and oral/manual automatisms are common. Focal to bilateral tonic clonic evolution (secondary generalization), if it occurs typically late in the seizure. The interictal EEG may show slowing (temporal intermittent rhythmic delta activity) and/or discharges in the anterior temporal channels (such as F7/F8). The ictal EEG is characterized by rhythmic alpha-theta or spikes. Postictal focal slowing (ipsilateral to the focus) is common. Figure 20.2 shows temporal intermittent rhythmic delta activity (TIRDA) while Figure 20.3 shows a mesial temporal lobe seizure.

2. Lateral temporal lobe epilepsy (LTLS, also called neocortical epilepsy) typically has auditory or vertiginous aura that precedes focal onset seizures with impaired awareness and behavioral arrest. Secondary generalization is more frequent and rapid compared to mesial temporal lobe seizures. The interictal EEG may show slowing and/or discharges in the mid-temporal or posterior channels (such as T7/T8). The ictal EEG shows rhythmic patterns with variable amplitudes and frequencies associated with rapid spread [5]. Figure 20.4 shows a lateral temporal lobe seizure.

Parietal Lobe Epilepsy: Parietal lobe epilepsy is typically characterized by focal nonmotor onset seizures which may be positive (paresthesia)/ negative(numbness) sensory phenomena. Disorientation, complex visual hallucinations, vertiginous, and visual illusions or disturbances of body

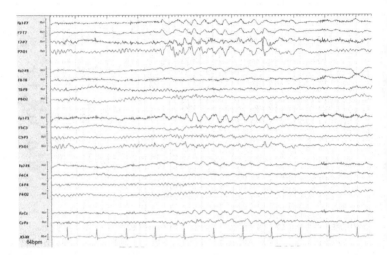

Figure 20.2 Fifty-year-old woman with mesial temporal sclerosis, left temporal intermittent rhythmic delta activity (TIRDA).

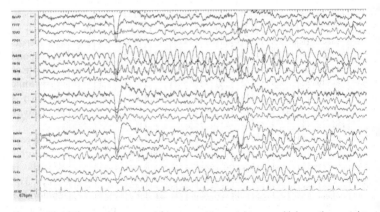

Figure 20.3 Twenty-three-year-old woman with mesial temporal lobe epilepsy, right anterior temporal sharp rhythmic theta activity at ictal onset of seizure.

image may occur along with receptive aphasias and ipsilateral or contralateral rotatory body movements. The interictal EEG may show abnormalities in the posterior channels, these can be precipitated by

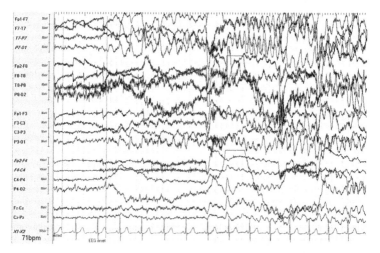

Figure 20.4 Twenty-eight-year-old woman with lateral temporal lobe epilepsy, left temporal sharp rhythmic delta-theta activity at ictal onset with rapid bilateral spread.

reflex sensory stimulation/touch. The ictal EEG is often unhelpful being normal or shows nonspecific slowing [6].

Occipital Lobe Epilepsy: Occipital lobe epilepsy is typically characterized by focal nonmotor onset seizures, which are often simple visual phenomena. Oculomotor features such as forced eye closure, eyelid flutter, eye deviation, and nystagmus also occur. The interictal EEG may show an asymmetric posterior-dominant alpha or photic responses and high-amplitude occipital spikes (Panayiotopoulos syndrome). The ictal EEG is characterized by occipital paroxysmal fast or rhythmic spike activity; lateralized or generalized ictal rhythms may also occur [7]. Figure 20.5 shows an occipital seizure.

Insular Epilepsy: The insula is an in-folded region of cortex located within the lateral sulcus that is sometimes referred to as a fifth lobe. Insular seizures are typically characterized by cervical-laryngeal discomfort (chocking), dyspnea, painful paresthesia, or temperature alterations, though they can mimic frontal, temporal, or parietal seizures. Interictal and ictal surface EEG is seldom useful given the deep location of seizure foci in this form of epilepsy [8].

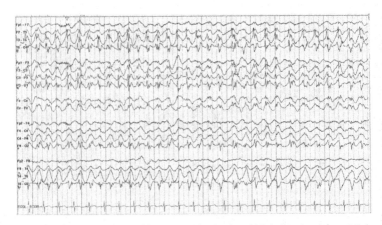

Figure 20.5 Nineteen-year-old woman with mitochondrial dysfunction, left occipital seizure (O1) with bilateral spread.

Generalized Epilepsy: Generalized epilepsies are characterized by generalized onset seizures types. Generalized ictal and interictal EEG abnormalities (generalized spike waves) are supportive, as is a positive family history. Generalized epilepsies are considered to have a genetic etiology though they aren't always inherited and may result from spontaneous mutations. Some authors use the term genetic generalized epilepsy in cases with strong inheritance and idiopathic generalized epilepsy (IGE) for those without it, however, these terms are used interchangeably. Generalized epilepsies are usually syndromic such as childhood absence epilepsy (CAE), juvenile absence epilepsy (JAE), or juvenile myoclonic epilepsy (JME).

Multifocal and Mixed Epilepsy (Focal and Generalized Epilepsy)

Multifocal epilepsies typically result from diffuse and symptomatic brain injuries such as global ischemia, encephalitis, or trauma. They are associated with multifocal discharges. Figure 20.6 shows multifocal discharges in a child with cerebral palsy.

Mixed epilepsies are characterized by both focal and generalized onset seizures and similar ictal and interictal EEG abnormalities. There are usually syndromic such as Dravet syndrome and Lennox–Gastaut syndrome. Common epilepsy syndromes are described in the following chapter (Chapter 21).

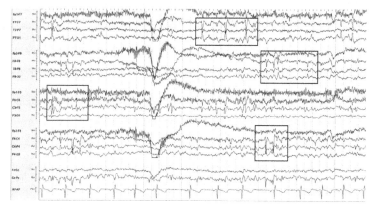

Figure 20.6 Six-year-old boy with cerebral palsy, multifocal spikes involving multiple channels (T7, P7, T8, C3, and C4).

Chapter Summary

1. Epilepsy is a disorder of recurrent unprovoked (or reflex) seizures; the key to diagnosing epilepsy is estimating the risk of recurrence.
2. Epilepsy may be diagnosed if a patient has two or more seizures at least 24 hours apart, a first-time seizure with factors that increase the risk of recurrence or an epilepsy syndrome.
3. When determining the type of epilepsy, first identify the seizure type(s), then the corresponding epilepsy type.
4. Consider if the epilepsy is potentially syndromic or nonsyndromic.
5. Consider the underlying etiology (structural, genetic, infectious, immune, or metabolic).
6. Focal epilepsies may be classified based on their region of onset, that is, frontal, temporal (mesial/lateral), parietal, occipital, and insular.
7. Ictal and interictal EEG findings vary with the type of focal epilepsy.

References

1. Fisher RS, Acevedo C, Arzimanoglou A, et al. ILAE official report: a practical clinical definition of epilepsy. *Epilepsia*. 2014 Apr;**55**(4):475–82.

2. Krumholz A, Wiebe S, Gronseth GS, et al. Evidence-based guideline: management of an unprovoked first seizure in adults: report of the Guideline Development

Subcommittee of the American Academy of Neurology and the American Epilepsy Society: evidence-based guideline. *Epilepsy Currents*. 2015 May;15(3):144–52.

3. Fisher RS, Cross JH, D'souza C, et al. Instruction manual for the ILAE 2017 operational classification of seizure types. *Epilepsia*. 2017 Apr;58(4):531–42.

4. McGonigal A, Chauvel P. Frontal lobe epilepsy: seizure semiology and presurgical evaluation. *Practical Neurology*. 2004 Oct 1;4(5):260–73.

5. Marks WJ Jr, Laxer KD. Semiology of temporal lobe seizures: value in lateralizing the seizure focus. *Epilepsia*. 1998 Jul;39(7):721–6.

6. Siegel AM, Williamson PD. Parietal lobe epilepsy. *Advances in Neurology*. 2000;84:189–99.

7. Williamson PD, Thadani VM, Darcey TM, et al. Occipital lobe epilepsy: clinical characteristics, seizure spread patterns, and results of surgery. *Annals of Neurology*. 1992 Jan;31(1):3–13.

8. Obaid S, Zerouali Y, Nguyen DK. Insular epilepsy: semiology and noninvasive investigations. *Journal of Clinical Neurophysiology*. 2017 Jul 1;34(4):315–23.

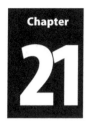

Epilepsy Syndromes

Epilepsy syndromes (electroclinical syndromes) are well-recognized group-ings of clinical (seizure types) and EEG features that occur together. Each syndrome typically shares a common age of onset, deficits (intellectual dys-function), treatment, and prognosis. Syndromes are classified based on their onset, epilepsy type (focal, generalized or mixed) and development of epileptic encephalopathy (disorder in which epileptic activity contributes to severe impairments in cognition and behavior) *.

Relatively benign syndromes are typically associated with focal, general-ized tonic clonic (GTC), typical absences, and myoclonic seizures. Epileptic encephalopathies are typically associated with atonic, tonic, atypical absences and epileptic spasms in addition to the above seizure types [1].

Epilepsy Syndromes

Neonatal Period
- benign neonatal convulsions
- early infantile epileptic encephalopathy (Ohtahara's syndrome) *
- early myoclonic encephalopathy (EME) *

Infancy
- benign infantile seizures
- epilepsy of infancy with migrating focal seizures (migrating partial seizures of infancy)
- myoclonic epilepsy in infancy
- infantile spasms (West syndrome) *
- myoclonic encephalopathy in nonprogressive disorders *

Childhood
- benign epilepsy with centrotemporal spikes (BECTS)
- early childhood onset occipital epilepsy (Panayiotopoulos syndrome)
- late childhood onset occipital epilepsy (Gastaut syndrome)
- childhood absence epilepsy (CAE)
- epilepsy with myoclonic absences (EMA)
- myoclonic-atonic/astatic epilepsy (Doose syndrome)

- generalized epilepsy with febrile seizures plus (GEFs plus)
- severe myoclonic epilepsy (Dravet syndrome) *
- epileptic encephalopathy with continuous spike and wave during sleep (CSWS) *
- Landau Kleffner syndrome (LKS) *
- Lennox–Gastaut syndrome (LGS) *

Adolescence and Adulthood
- autosomal-dominant nocturnal frontal lobe epilepsy (ADNFLE)
- autosomal-dominant temporal lobe epilepsy with auditory features (ADTLE)
- familial temporal lobe epilepsies
- juvenile absence epilepsy (JAE)
- juvenile myoclonic epilepsy (JME)
- epilepsy with generalized tonic clonic seizures alone (EGTCA)
- progressive myoclonic epilepsies (PME)

Any Age (Less Age Specific)
- familial focal epilepsy with variable foci (FFEVF)
- reflex epilepsies

Some epilepsy disorders may not be syndromic but nevertheless share recognizable features (distinctive constellations), these include Rasmussen's syndrome, gelastic seizures with hypothalamic hamartoma (HH), and hemi convulsion-hemiplegia epilepsy (HHE).

The remainder of this chapter discusses the EEG features of common epilepsy syndromes.

Neonatal Syndromes

Benign Neonatal Convulsions

These are also called benign idiopathic neonatal seizures or fifth day fits. They occur in the first week of life as unifocal clonic seizures with apnea/cyanosis. There are no neurodevelopmental deficits. The etiology is believed to be genetic such as potassium channel defects. Typically resolve by the second week (self-limited) though some develop seizures in later life. Interictal EEG may be normal or show "theta pointu alternant" which are bursts of focal, nonreactive theta activity intermixed with multifocal sharp waves that alternate between hemisphere [2].

Early Infantile Epileptic Encephalopathy (Otohara Syndrome)

This is an epileptic encephalopathy that typically occurs within the first three months of life. It is characterized by tonic seizures, infantile spasms, and

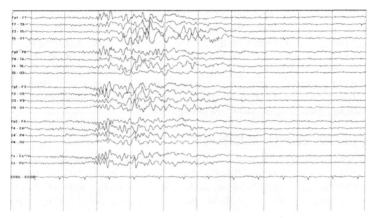

Figure 21.1 One-month-old boy with porencephaly, burst-suppression pattern.

myoclonic seizures. Structural etiologies (such as cortical dysplasia) are common. The prognosis is usually poor with high mortality. Interictal EEG shows burst-suppression regardless of clinical state as shown in Figure 21.1 [3].

Early Myoclonic Encephalopathy (EME)

This is an epileptic encephalopathy typically occurs within the first month of life. It is characterized by myoclonic seizures involving face or limbs, focal seizures, and tonic spams. Metabolic etiologies (such as nonketotic hyperglycinemia/pyridoxine deficiency) are common. The prognosis is poor with high mortality. Interictal EEG shows burst-suppression, may be only during sleep. At 3–5 months of age, the waking EEG is replaced by hypsarrhythmia, this reverts to burst-suppression around 2–3 years of age [3].

Infantile Syndromes

Benign Infantile Seizures

Both familial and nonfamilial forms exist, nonfamilial forms. They typically occur between 3 months to 3 years of life (nonfamilial forms have later onsets) with focal clonic seizures of the head, face, and limbs that may generalize. Normal Neurodevelopment. Self-limited with a good prognosis. Interictal EEG is normal. Ictal EEG shows focal onset temporal/posterior seizures [4].

Epilepsy of Infancy with Migrating Focal Seizures

These were previously called migrating partial seizures of infancy. Typical onset is around 3 months of age with sporadic focal motor seizures. These often cluster and show bilateral spread. Neurodevelopment is normal at presentation but declines. Genetic etiologies (such as sodium and potassium channel defects) are common. Poor prognosis with high mortality. Interictal EEG shows multifocal slowing with disruption of sleep architecture. Ictal EEG shows multifocal or migrating seizure onsets [5].

Myoclonic Epilepsy in Infancy

This is the earliest form of idiopathic generalized epilepsy occurring between 3 months to 3 years of age. Bilateral myoclonic jerks, head drops, or truncal spasms may also occur. Seizures may be reflexive to auditory or other stimuli. Neurodevelopment is normal. Self-limited with good prognosis. Jerks are associated with fast generalized, irregular spike, or polyspikes discharges as shown in Figure 21.2 [6].

Infantile Spasms (West Syndrome)

West syndrome is a triad of spasms, hypsarrhythmia on EEG, and developmental delay. The typical onset is around 4 to 8 months of age with clusters of flexor or extensor spasms several times a day. Structural (such as tuberous sclerosis), genetic, metabolic, and infectious etiologies are common. Epileptic encephalopathy with a poor prognosis. Hypsarrhythmia refers to continuous,

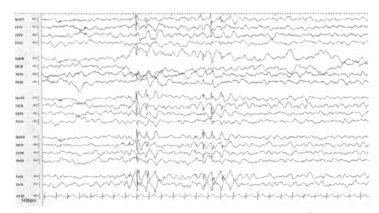

Figure 21.2 Twelve-month-old boy with myoclonic epilepsy in infancy, generalized 3 Hz discharges.

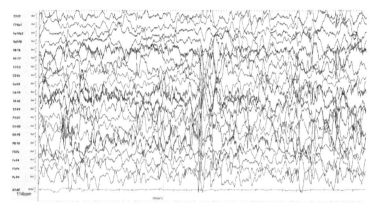

Figure 21.3 Nine-month-old boy with West syndrome, hypsarrhythmia (sensitivity 10 uV).

arrhythmic, high-amplitude, asynchronous delta activity with multifocal independent discharges (chaotic) on interictal EEG as shown in Figure 21.3. Diffuse suppressions are seen during spasms as shown in Chapter 19, Figure 19.6 [3,7].

Myoclonic Encephalopathy in Nonprogressive Disorders

This is a rare disorder with typical onset in the first year of life and is characterized by continuous myoclonic jerking in the absence of a progressive encephalopathy. Genetic etiology such as Angelman syndrome are common. Epileptic encephalopathy with poor prognosis. Interictal EEG shows diffuse theta-delta or delta with spikes as shown in Figure 21.4 [3].

Childhood Syndromes

Benign Epilepsy with Centrotemporal Spikes (BECTS)

This is also called Rolandic epilepsy and is the most common focal epilepsy of childhood. Typically occur around 7 to 10 years of age with unilateral or bilateral, sensory or motor seizures that are characterized by oropharyngeal manifestations (numbness, paresthesia, gurgling, grunting, or drooling) or speech arrest. May spread to face and hand with secondary generalization. Seizures are commonly nocturnal. Neurodevelopmentally normal, though occasional concerns with language may occur. The etiology is believed to be genetic. Good prognosis with most patients remitting before age 16. Interictal EEG typically shows centrotemporal spikes (CTS) these are clusters of high-amplitude, sharp and slow-wave

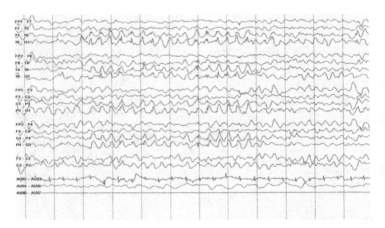

Figure 21.4 Twelve-month-old girl with Angelman's syndrome, occipital-predominant delta with spikes.

discharges that that phase reverse over central (C3-C4), temporal, or parietal regions on a longitudinal bipolar montage. They can be amplified during sleep and sometimes with somatosensory stimulation. They are usually bilateral and asymmetric with characteristic horizontal dipoles (surface negative over the central region but simultaneously positive over the frontal region). Slowing after spikes may suggest a greater challenge with seizure control. Decrease of spikes in sleep, fast/polyspikes, and burst-suppression after spikes may suggest alternative diagnosis. Ictal EEG is variable and may show evolving discharges, low-voltage fast rhythmic activity, or rhythmic theta. Figure 21.5 shows centro-temporal spikes and Figure 21.6 shows their characteristic horizontal dipole on referential montage [8].

Early Childhood Onset Occipital Epilepsy (Panayiotopoulos Syndrome)

Typically occurs between 3 to 6 years of age with agitation, headache and autonomic symptoms (such as a nausea, vomiting, pallor, and cyanosis) leading to a prolonged hemiclonic or generalized motor seizure. Autonomic status epilepticus may occur. Seizures are infrequent and may not need treatment. Neurodevelopmentally normal. Self-limited epilepsy with good prognosis. Interictal EEG shows salvos of bilateral, independent, occipital spikes, especially in sleep. Figure 21.7 shows occipital spikes in Panayiotopoulos syndrome [9].

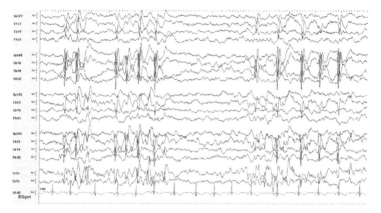

Figure 21.5 Seven-year-old girl with Rolandic epilepsy, centrotemporal spikes with a right temporal predominance (sensitivity 20 uV).

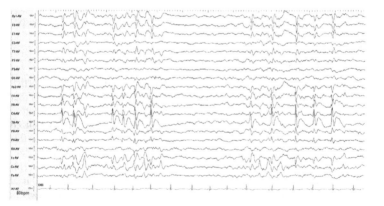

Figure 21.6 Same patient as in Figure 21.5, horizontal dipole on referential montage (sensitivity 20 uV).

Late Childhood Onset Occipital Epilepsy (Gastaut Syndrome)

Typically occurs between 8 and 11 years of age with elementary visual auras or visual field cuts leading to a focal seizure with rare secondary generalization. Headaches occur but autonomic symptoms are uncommon. Seizures are more frequent compared to Panayiotopoulos syndrome, needing treatment.

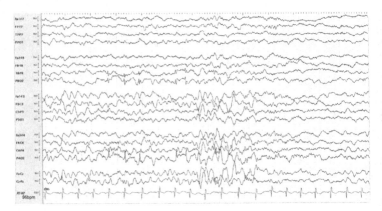

Figure 21.7 Three-year-old girl with Panayiotopoulos syndrome, right occipital spikes (sensitivity 10 uV).

Neurodevelopmentally normal. Self-limited epilepsy with good prognosis. Interictal EEG shows bilateral, independent, occipital spikes in salvos, especially with sleep and eye closure [9].

Childhood Absence Epilepsy (CAE)

Begins in the preschool (3 to 10 years) with typical absences (staring spells). These are characterized by transient unresponsiveness and event amnesia that may occur several times a day. Seizures can be provoked by hyperventilation and often have motor automatisms. Minority have at least one generalized tonic clonic seizure. Genetic etiologies are thought to be responsible for this syndrome. In those with an early onset Glucose Transporter (GLUT-1) deficiency should be considered. Neurodevelopmentally normal. Self-limited epilepsy but often poor social outcomes. Interictal EEG is typically normal. Ictal EEG shows regular 3 Hz generalized spike and wave pattern as shown in Figure 21.8. Rarely photosensitive [10].

Epilepsy with Myoclonic Absences (EMA)

Typical onset occurs around 5 to 12 years of age with myoclonic absences. These are brief absences (10 to 60 s) with axial hypertonia. Drop attacks or generalized tonic clonic seizures may also occur. Neurodevelopmental delay/decline is common. Both structural or genetic etiologies may be responsible. The prognosis is variable but cognitive impairment and epilepsy often persist into adulthood. Interictal EEG may be normal or show generalized discharges.

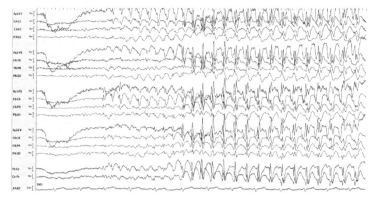

Figure 21.8 Eight-year-old boy with CAE, typical absences with 3 Hz generalized spike and wave discharges.

Ictal EEG shows regular 3 Hz generalized spike and wave discharges typically provoked by hyperventilation or photic stimulation [11].

Myoclonic-Atonic/astatic Epilepsy (Doose Syndrome)

Typically occurs around 1 to 5 years of age with acute onset of atonic, absence, and myoclonic seizures in a previously normal child. There may be a family history of epilepsy. Cognitive decline occurs and seizures are refractory to medications. Interictal EEG may be normal or show a central rhythmic theta. Ictal EEG (myoclonic-atonic seizure) shows 2–4 Hz generalized spike wave discharges as shown in Figure 21.9 [12].

Generalized Epilepsy with Febrile Seizures Plus (GEFS Plus)

Febrile seizures persist beyond 6 years of age or occur before six months. There is a strong family history of generalized epilepsy and/or febrile seizures. Nonfebrile seizures may occur. The etiology is thought to be secondary to a sodium channel related gene defect (SCN1A). Normal neurodevelopment. Self-limited, usually remits before puberty. Interictal EEG is normal. Ictal EEG depends on the seizure type [13].

Severe Myoclonic Epilepsy (Dravet Syndrome)

Epileptic encephalopathy with a typical onset before 2 years of age, heralded by a prolonged febrile seizure (hemi convulsion). These are followed by focal afebrile seizures (switch sides), myoclonus, and later multiple seizure types

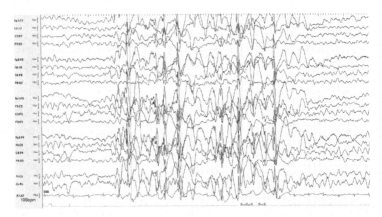

Figure 21.9 Three-year-old boy with Doose syndrome (myoclonic astatic epilepsy), 3 to 2.5 Hz generalized spike and wave discharges (sensitivity 20 uV).

often precipitated by fever. Genetic etiology (SCN1A defect) is responsible. Neurodevelopment may be normal at presentation, but progressively declines. Seizures are refractory and the prognosis is poor. Interictal EEG is initially normal, then deteriorates, and generalized discharges appear as shown in Figure 21.10 [3].

Epileptic Encephalopathy with Continuous Spike and Wave during Sleep (CSWS)

This is also called electrical status epilepticus during slow-wave sleep (ESES). Onset occurs between ages 5 to 10 years of age with seizures followed by cognitive decline that persists despite seizure resolution. Both structural and genetic etiologies may be responsible. EEG shows generalized discharges, marked sleep activation comprising greater than 85% of non–rapid eye movement (NREM) sleep as shown in Figure 21.11. Discharges significantly reduce in REM sleep. Typically, poor prognosis with severe behavioral and intellectual dysfunction [3].

Landau Kleffner Syndrome (LKS)

Typically, onset occurs between 3 to 6 years of age with verbal auditory aphasia, expressive aphasia, and focal seizures follow. Genetic (GRIN2A mutation) or autoimmune etiologies may be responsible. Seizures remit but language/cognitive deficits worsen (epileptic encephalopathy). EEG is like ESES but may have focal/multifocal spikes [3].

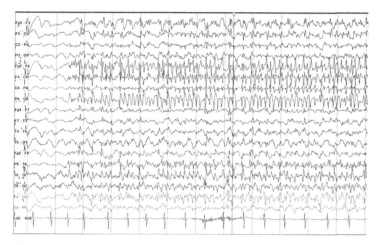

Figure 21.10 Twelve-month-old boy with Dravet syndrome (severe myoclonic epilepsy), background slowing, and abundant generalized discharges.

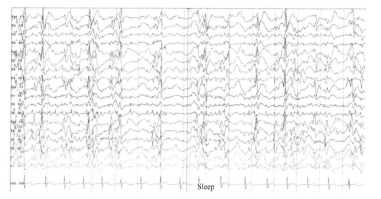

Figure 21.11 Seven-year-old girl with intellectual disability, continuous generalized discharges during NREM sleep.

Lennox–Gastaut Syndrome (LGS)

This is an epileptic encephalopathy with onset between 1 to 10 years of age. Multiple seizure types including tonic, atypical absences, and atonic

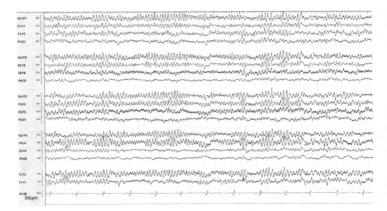

Figure 21.12 Thirty-one-year-old woman with LGS, generalized bursts of 10 Hz activity during NREM sleep.

seizures are characteristic. Myoclonic, focal, and generalized tonic clonic seizures also occur. In some, infantile spasms precede the onset of LGS. Structural, postinfectious, or genetic etiologies are usually responsible. The prognosis is poor with cognitive dysfunction, refractory epilepsy, and status epilepticus. Interictal EEG shows slow background with bursts of irregular generalized slow spike and wave discharges that are accentuated during NREM sleep as shown in Chapter 14, Figure 14.11. Generalized fast bursts (10 Hz) during NREM sleep also occur (Figure 21.12). Ictal EEG depends on seizure type, may show generalized discharge followed by a burst of diffuse fast activity (tonic seizures), generalized slow spike and wave discharges (atypical absences), polyspikes or diffuse fast activity (atonic or myoclonic seizures) as previously described in Chapter 19 [3,12].

Adolescent and Adult Syndromes

Autosomal-Dominant Nocturnal Frontal Lobe Epilepsy (ADNFLE)

Typically occurs around 12 years of age with nocturnal hyperkinetic seizures that cluster. Retained awareness and aura are common. Normal neurodevelopment. Genetic etiologies (nicotinic cholinergic receptor defects) are responsible. Interictal EEG is normal. Ictal EEG shows bifrontal onsets [14].

Autosomal-Dominant Temporal Lobe Epilepsy with Auditory Features (ADTLE)

This is also called autosomal-dominant lateral temporal lobe epilepsy. The onset usually occurs in the first or second decade of life, but may be later. Lateral temporal lobe seizures with prominent ictal auditory symptoms and/or receptive aphasia occur. Normal neurodevelopment. Genetic etiologies (LGI1 defect) are responsible. Interictal EEG is normal. Ictal EEG shows lateral temporal lobe onset. Pharmacoresponsive epilepsy with good prognosis [15].

Familial Mesial Temporal Lobe Epilepsies (FMTLE)

Numerous relatively benign, familial, mesial temporal lobe epilepsies occur typically in the first or second decade of life and follow a mild clinical course that may remit. Three main presentations include those without febrile seizures/hippocampal sclerosis (prominent autonomic and psychic aura), those with hippocampal sclerosis (prominent automatisms and postictal changes) and those with febrile seizures. Hippocampal sclerosis may occur in asymptomatic family members [16].

Juvenile Absence Epilepsy (JAE)

Typical onset is around 10 to 12 years of age with infrequent absences followed by generalized tonic clonic seizures. Cognitive dysfunction may occur. Variable prognosis, typically pharmacoresponsive but may not remit with age. Interictal EEG shows 3–6 Hz generalized discharges not typically provoked by hyperventilation (Figure 21.13) [10].

Juvenile Myoclonic Epilepsy (JME)

Most common genetic generalized epilepsies with typical onset between ages 12 to 20 years. Classically presents with morning myoclonus, generalized tonic clonic seizures, and less commonly absences. Seizure triggers include sleep deprivation, alcohol, and photic stimulation. Good prognosis with normal cognition and pharmacoresponsive seizures but typically doesn't resolve with age. EEG shows 4–6 Hz (fast) generalized discharges (Figure 21.14) [10].

Epilepsy with Generalized Tonic Clonic Seizures Alone

Typically occur between 10 to 25 years with generalized tonic clonic seizures upon awakening. Some may have nocturnal seizures. Sleep deprivation, alcohol, and photosensitivity are common triggers. Cognition is normal. Interictal EEG shows generalized discharges [10].

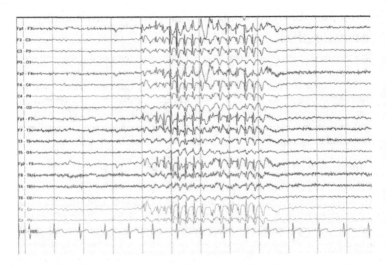

Figure 21.13 Ten-year-old boy with JAE, generalized 4 Hz spike, and wave discharges.

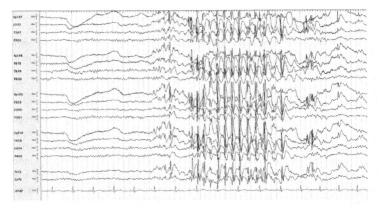

Figure 21.14 Twelve-year-old boy with JME, generalized 4 Hz spike, and wave discharges (sensitivity 20 uV).

Progressive Myoclonic Epilepsies

These are a manifestation of underlying neurometabolic and neurodegenerative diseases. They are characterized by cognitive decline (epileptic encephalopathy) and intractable myoclonus. Unvericht–Lundborg syndrome (UVL), Lafora body disease, and neuronal ceroid lipofuscinosis (NCL) are common causes. EEG typically shows a deteriorated background, multifocal epileptic discharges, and photosensitivity with giant evoked potentials. Poor prognosis with high mortality [3].

Less Age-Specific Syndromes and Other Constellations

Familial Focal Epilepsy with Variable Foci (FFEVF)

Typically occurs in the first or second decade of life and is characterized by focal onset seizures from different cortical regions. Variable neurodevelopmental outcomes including autism may occur. Genetic etiology (DEPDC5 gene defect on chromosome 22). EEG findings are variable [17].

Progressive Unilateral Encephalopathy of Childhood (Rasmussen's Syndrome)

Typically occurs between 3 and 14 years of age with focal seizures (often epilepsia partialis continua) and other unilateral deficits. There is progressive unihemispheric cortical atrophy on neuroimaging. Normal development at onset but later declines. Histopathology shows a T-cell mediated encephalitis (autoimmune etiology) with microglial nodules and reactive astrogliosis. Interictal EEG shows unihemispheric slowing and epileptic discharges [18].

Gelastic Seizures with Hypothalamic Hamartoma (HH)

Hypothalamic hamartomas are intrinsically epileptogenic due to GABA neurons. They classically present with gelastic seizures (emotionless laughter). Other seizures including dacrystic seizures (crying) may occur. Precocious puberty, behavioral problems, and cognitive dysfunction are common. Interictal and ictal EEG may be normal [19].

Hemi Convulsion-Hemiplegia Epilepsy (HHE)

This is an uncommon form of epilepsy that occurs in late infancy or toddlers and is characterized by prolonged focal or generalized status epilepticus followed by hemiplegia. May be idiopathic or symptomatic due to other pathology (such as stroke, infection, or trauma) [20].

Reflex Epilepsies

Multiple reflex epilepsies have been identified based on the triggering stimulus such as visual/photosensitivity, reading, music, tactile, hot water, and others.

Chapter Summary

Common age-dependent epilepsy syndromes

Syndrome	Epilepsy	Seizures	EEG (interictal)	Cognitive impairment	Course
Neonatal syndromes					
Benign neonatal convulsions	Focal	Focal (apneic)	Theta pointu alternant	None	Self-limited
Otohara syndrome	Epileptic encephalopathy	Tonic	Burst-suppression	Severe	Poor prognosis
Early myoclonic encephalopathy	Epileptic encephalopathy	Myoclonic	Burst-suppression	Severe	Poor prognosis
Infantile syndromes					
Benign infantile seizures	Focal	Focal clonic	Normal	None	Self-limited
Epilepsy of infancy with migrating focal seizures	Multifocal	Clusters of focal motor	Multifocal or migrating patterns	Initially normal, then declines	Poor prognosis
Myoclonic epilepsy in infancy	Generalized (IGE)	Myoclonus, head drops, truncal spams	1–3 Hz generalized discharges	None	Self-limited
West syndrome	Epileptic encephalopathy	Clusters of flexor or extensor spasm	Hypsarrhythmia	Severe	Poor prognosis
Myoclonic encephalopathy in nonprogressive disorders	Epileptic encephalopathy	Myoclonus	Diffuse theta or delta with spikes	Severe	Poor prognosis
Childhood syndromes					
Benign epilepsy with centrotemporal spikes	Focal (Rolandic)	Oropharyngeal, speech or autonomic	Centrotemporal spikes	None	Self-limited

(cont.)

Syndrome	Epilepsy	Seizures	EEG (interictal)	Cognitive impairment	Course
Panayiotopoulos syndrome	Focal occipital	Autonomic, focal motor	Occipital spikes	None	Self-limited
Gastaut syndrome	Focal occipital	Visual, focal motor	Occipital spikes	None	Self-limited
Childhood absence epilepsy	Generalized (IGE)	Typical absences	GSW (3 Hz)	None	Self-limited
Epilepsy with myoclonic absences	Generalized (IGE)	Absences with axial hypertonia	GSW (3 Hz)	Moderate	Variable
Doose syndrome	Generalized (IGE)	Atonic, absences and myoclonic	Central rhythmic theta, GSW (2–4 Hz)	Moderate	Poor prognosis
GEF plus	Generalized	Febrile and afebrile seizures	Normal	None	Self-limited
Dravet syndrome	Epileptic encephalopathy	Febrile and afebrile seizures, other types	Slowing, generalized discharges	Initially normal, then severe decline	Poor prognosis
CSWS	Epileptic encephalopathy	Generalized	Generalized discharges, 85% of NREM sleep	Severe	Poor prognosis
LKS	Epileptic encephalopathy	Focal	as above	Language	Poor prognosis
LGS	Epileptic encephalopathy	Tonic, atypical absences, atonic and others	Slow spike and wave (2–2.5 Hz)	Severe	Poor prognosis
Adolescent and adult syndromes					
ADNFLE	Focal	Hyperkinetic	Normal	None	Pharmaco-responsive

(cont.)

Syndrome	Epilepsy	Seizures	EEG (interictal)	Cognitive impairment	Course
ADTLE	Focal	Auditory aura, receptive aphasia	Normal	None	Pharmaco-responsive
FMTLE	Focal	Autonomic, psychic aura	Normal	None	Pharmaco-responsive
JAE	Generalized (IGE)	Infrequent absences, GTCs	Generalized discharges (3.5–6 Hz)	Variable	Variable
JME	Generalized (IGE)	Myoclonus, GTCs, rare absences	Generalized discharges (4–6 Hz)	None	Pharmaco-responsive
Epilepsy with generalized tonic clonic seizures alone	Generalized (IGE)	GTC	Generalized discharges	None	Pharmaco-responsive
PME	Epileptic encephalo-pathy	Myoclonus	Giant photic evoked potentials	Severe	Poor prognosis

References

1. Scheffer IE, Berkovic S, Capovilla G, et al. ILAE classification of the epilepsies: position paper of the ILAE Commission for Classification and Terminology. *Epilepsia*. 2017 Apr;**58**(4):512–21.

2. Miles DK, Holmes GL. Benign neonatal seizures. *Journal of Clinical Neurophysiology*. 1990 Jul;7(3):369–79.

3. Donat JF. Topical review article: the age-dependent epileptic encephalopathies. *Journal of Child Neurology*. 1992 Jan;7(1):7–21.

4. Vigevano F. Benign familial infantile seizures. *Brain and Development*. 2005 Apr 1;27(3):172–7.

5. Caraballo RH, Fontana E, Darra F, et al. Migrating focal seizures in infancy: analysis of the electroclinical patterns in 17 patients. *Journal of Child Neurology*. 2008 May;23(5):497–506.

6. Dravet C, Bureau M. Benign myoclonic epilepsy in infancy. *Epileptic Syndromes in Infancy, Childhood and Adolescence*. 2005;4:77–88.

7. Quigg M. *EEG pearls*. Mosby Elsevier, New York; 2006.

8. Donald Shields W, Carter Snead O III. Benign epilepsy with centrotemporal spikes. *Epilepsia*. 2009 Sep;**50**:10–15.

9. Yalçin AD, Kaymaz A, Forta H. Childhood occipital epilepsy: seizure manifestations and electroencephalographic features. *Brain and Development*. 1997 Sep 1;**19**(6):408–13.

10. Mattson RH. Overview: idiopathic generalized epilepsies. *Epilepsia*. 2003 Mar;**44**:2–6.

11. Tassinari CA, Rubboli G, Gardella EL, Michelucci RO. Epilepsy with myoclonic absences. *Epilepsy in Children*. 2004 Feb;**27**:189–94.

12. Stephani U. The natural history of myoclonic astatic epilepsy (Doose syndrome) and Lennox-Gastaut syndrome. *Epilepsia*. 2006 Nov;**47**:53–5.

13. Camfield P, Camfield C. Febrile seizures and genetic epilepsy with febrile seizures plus (GEFS+). *Epileptic Disorders*. 2015 Jun;**17**(2):124–33.

14. Bertrand D, Picard F, Le Hellard S, et al. How mutations in the nAChRs can cause ADNFLE epilepsy. *Epilepsia*. 2002 Jun;**43**:112–22.

15. Michelucci R, Pasini E, Nobile C. Lateral temporal lobe epilepsies: clinical and genetic features. *Epilepsia*. 2009 May;**50**:52–4.

16. Gambardella A, Labate A, Giallonardo A, Aguglia U. Familial mesial temporal lobe epilepsies: clinical and genetic features. *Epilepsia*. 2009 May;**50**:55–7.

17. Dibbens LM, De Vries B, Donatello S, et al. Mutations in DEPDC5 cause familial focal epilepsy with variable foci. *Nature Genetics*. 2013 May;**45**(5):546.

18. Vining EP, Freeman JM, Brandt J, Carson BS, Uematsu S. Progressive unilateral encephalopathy of childhood (Rasmussen's syndrome): a reappraisal. *Epilepsia*. 1993 Jul;**34**(4):639–50.

19. Arroyo S, Lesser RP, Gordon B, et al. Mirth, laughter and gelastic seizures. *Brain*. 1993 Aug 1;**116**(4):757–80.

20. Gastaut H, Poirier F, Payan H, Salamon G, Toga M, Vigouroux MH. HHE syndrome hemiconvulsions, hemiplegia, epilepsy. *Epilepsia*. 1959 Jan;**1**(1–5):418–47.

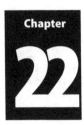

Focal Dysfunction (Lesions)

A structural lesion such as an infarction, hemorrhage, tumor, or abscess causes local cerebral dysfunction and resultant EEG abnormalities. The EEG is a poorly sensitive and specific test to detect structural brain lesions compared to advanced neuroimaging techniques such as magnetic resonance imaging (MRI) but has a key role in determining the lesion's functional significance (such as epileptogenicity) [1]. Additionally, the EEG can determine physiologic cerebral dysfunction, such as postictal state or hypoperfusion, which are often reversible and without corresponding structural correlate on neuroimaging. The role of the reader is to detect if focal dysfunction is present and estimate its potential severity, etiology (structural or functional), and epileptogenicity.

Basic Approach to Focal Cerebral Dysfunction on EEG

1. detection
2. estimate severity
3. estimate if structural (fixed) or functional (reversible) underlying etiology
4. estimate potential for seizures (epileptogenicity)

Detecting Focal Cerebral Dysfunction

Two key EEG features indicate the presence of focal dysfunction:

1. *Disruption of background activity in the ipsilateral hemisphere*: During wakefulness, there may be asymmetric slowing, amplitude attenuation, or decreased reactivity of the posterior-dominant rhythm (Bancaud's phenomena refers to the persistence of alpha during eye opening on the side of hemispheric dysfunction). Anterior faster frequencies (beta) may also be asymmetrically decreased. During drowsiness/sleep, there may be an asymmetric disruption of sleep architecture. Asymmetries in photic driving response and/or hyperventilation build-up may be elicited during activation procedures.
2. *Emergence of focal slowing (delta or theta waves)*: Focal abnormalities indicate local cerebral dysfunction. Focal slowing (theta or delta waves) is the most common abnormality. It may occur sporadically or in abundance and is thought to be caused by the disruption of cortical connections in the cerebral white matter [2].

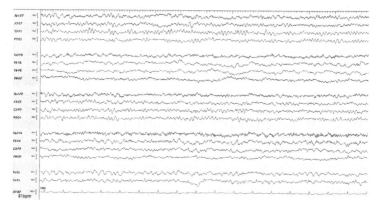

Figure 22.1 Sixty-seven-year-old woman with glioblastoma, right hemispheric dysfunction that is maximal over the temporal region.

Figure 22.1 shows right hemispheric dysfunction worse over the temporal region and characterized by disruption of the normal background and polymorphic slowing.

Estimating Severity

Nonspecific electrographic markers of severity include the abundance of focal slowing in a record, attenuation of amplitude, increased slower frequencies, and the loss of reactivity to external stimulation or state change (usually recorded by the technologist). Milder forms of focal dysfunction may be accentuated during drowsiness. Some sporadic subtle temporal slowing in the elderly is not uncommon during drowsiness and may not have any clinical significance.

Structural (Fixed) versus Physiologic (Reversible) Focal Dysfunction

Reactive, intermittent (sporadic or bursts), or fluctuating slowing may indicate physiological dysfunction such as transient hypoperfusion (vasospasm or hemiplegic migraines) or a postictal state as shown in Chapter 14, Figure 14.14. These abnormalities are reversible and disappear on repeat recordings. There may not be any associated abnormalities on neuroimaging.

Structural (fixed) lesions are typically associated with abundant (often continuous) focal mixed polymorphic theta and delta slowing that does not react (alter or improve) to external stimulation or state change (arousal) as shown in Chapter 14, Figure 14.15.

These features, however, are neither sensitive nor specific.

Potential Epileptogenicity

Focal intermittent rhythmic (monomorphic) delta activity such as lateralized rhythmic delta activity (LRDA) of which temporal intermittent rhythmic delta activity (TIRDA) is a subtype are considered an epileptogenic abnormality (despite lacking sharp morphology) due to increased association with epileptic seizures as shown in Chapter 15, Figure 15.4.

Focal sporadic (sharps/spikes) or periodic (LPDs) epileptic discharges may also occur. Figure 22.2 shows continuous polymorphic delta slowing and paracentral periodic discharges over the left hemisphere.

A breach effect from an overlying skull defect (such as a craniotomy) may cause enhancement of amplitudes and sharpness that make the underlying cortical activity appear "epileptiform" as shown in Figure 22.3, caution should be exercised when interpreting sharp waves through a breach effect to avoid overcall. The technologist must note the location of skull defects.

Note that dysfunction may occur independently over both hemispheres as shown in Figure 22.4 (multifocal dysfunction). Focal dysfunction may also occur in the setting of diffuse cerebral dysfunction (encephalopathy) [3].

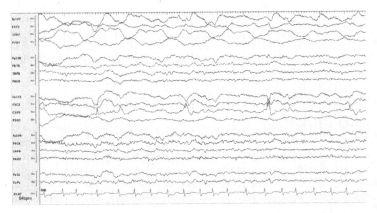

Figure 22.2 Sixty-three-year-old man with a left hemispheric stroke, predominant left hemispheric dysfunction, and cortical irritability. Additionally, there is evidence of a mild encephalopathy.

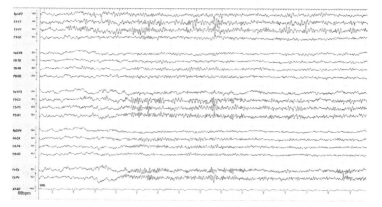

Figure 22.3 Sixty-four-year-old man with a craniotomy for subdural hematoma, left hemispheric breach effect.

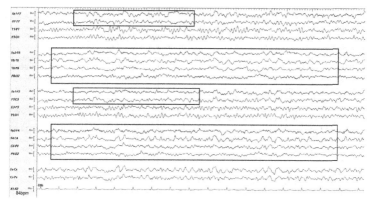

Figure 22.4 Same patient as in Figure 22.1, left frontal and prominent right hemispheric dysfunction.

Chapter Summary

1. The EEG is poorly sensitive and specific to detect lesions compared to neuroimaging; its practical use is to determine the functional consequence of the lesion.

2. Focal dysfunction (physiologic) may occur without an associated neuroimaging abnormality. Postictal states and hypoperfusion are examples of physiologic dysfunction, these are often reversible (disappear on repeat testing).

3. Focal dysfunction causes disruption of the ipsilateral hemispheric background architecture (wakefulness and sleep), asymmetric responses on activation procedures, and focal slowing.

4. Severity of the focal dysfunction may be estimated based on the abundance of focal slowing, attenuation of amplitude, and loss of reactivity.

5. Sporadic, intermittent, or fluctuating focal slowing that is reactive to external stimulation or endogenous state changes (such as arousal) may indicate physiological dysfunction.

6. Focal intermittent rhythmic (monomorphic) delta activity such as lateralized rhythmic delta activity (LRDA), specifically indicates epileptogenicity. It should be treated like an epileptic discharge despite the lack of a sharpness. Look for epileptic discharges that may accompany focal slowing.

7. Focal slowing may occur in isolation, bilaterally, or in the setting of diffuse cerebral dysfunction.

References

1. Noh BH, Berg AT, Nordli DR Jr. Concordance of MRI lesions and EEG focal slowing in children with nonsyndromic epilepsy. *Epilepsia*. 2013 Mar;54(3):455–60.

2. Britton JW, Frey LC, Hopp JL, et al. Electroencephalography (EEG): *an* introductory text and atlas of normal and abnormal findings in adults, children, and infants. American Epilepsy Society, Chicago; 2016.

3. Gaspard N, Manganas L, Rampal N, Petroff OA, Hirsch LJ. Similarity of lateralized rhythmic delta activity to periodic lateralized epileptiform discharges in critically ill patients. *JAMA Neurology*. 2013 Oct 1;70(10):1288–95.

Chapter 23

Global Dysfunction (Encephalopathy)

Altered mentation (encephalopathy), typically is a consequence of impaired functioning of both cerebral hemispheres and/or the brainstem (global dysfunction). Worsening encephalopathy may result in coma which is a deep and prolonged state of unconsciousness characterized by unresponsiveness to external stimuli, absence of sleep-wake cycles, and the lack of any voluntary actions [1].

The EEG is exquisitely sensitive to global cerebral dysfunction but is poorly specific to etiology. Multiple etiologies of encephalopathy may lead to similar electrographic patterns but have different prognosis. These patterns are typically abnormalities of background (Chapter 10) and repetitive abnormalities of foreground (Chapter 15). Less commonly, repetitive patterns represent ictal activity that contributes to the encephalopathic state (nonconvulsive status epilepticus) [2].

Occasionally, an EEG may appear normal in comatose individuals suggesting psychogenic coma or a locked-in state [3]. A handful of "classic" EEG presentations exist that may suggest a specific cause of encephalopathy, these are described in the later part of this chapter.

The reader's basic approach should be like that described for a focal lesion:

1. make diagnosis;
2. estimate severity;
3. identify any repetitive patterns and understand their implications;
4. identify nonconvulsive status epilepticus (NCSE).

Diagnosing Encephalopathy on EEG

Encephalopathy, which is synonymous with diffuse, global, or bilateral hemispheric dysfunction, is a common electrographic diagnosis in those with altered mentation. The three cardinal features of an encephalopathic EEG include (1) background slowing, (2) attenuation/discontinuity, and (3) decreased reactivity. In the initial stages of encephalopathy, there is slowing of the posterior-dominant rhythm (differentiate this from excessive drowsiness, where the PDR is brief but reactive and within alpha range), the background

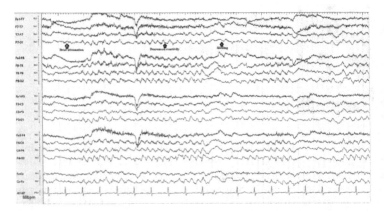

Figure 23.1 Fifty-two-year old man with confusion, early encephalopathic changes on EEG.

amplitude may be increased with emergence of theta and delta activities but later attenuates, and there is paradoxical or decreased reactivity to both endogenous state changes (such as arousals) or external stimulation. Paradoxical alpha refers to the emergence of an occipital alpha with eye opening and is typical of early encephalopathy [4].

Figure 23.1 shows early encephalopathy with emergence of diffuse slowing, brief periods of attenuation, and decreased reactivity of the background.

Estimating Severity

Progressive deterioration in the level of consciousness is typically associated with background slowing; there is emergence of theta and delta activities which may completely replace the normal background in more severe forms (Figure 23.2). Initially, there may be an increase in the background amplitude (voltage), but with worsening cerebral dysfunction, there is attenuation and then suppression of cerebral activity resulting in discontinuity. Burst suppression or even complete electrocerebral silence may be seen in the most severe forms. The progression of discontinuity is shown in Chapter 10, Figures 10.3, 10.4, and 10.5.

Loss of reactivity (and variability) is another important electrographic marker of severity. The loss of reactivity may be assessed by the technologist in a graded manner using increasing levels of stimulation. The clinical and electrographic response along with the specific stimulation should be recorded in real time.

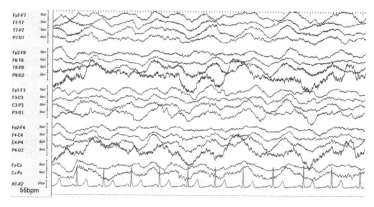

Figure 23.2 Same patient as in Figure 23.1, diffuse high-amplitude delta slowing with progression on encephalopathy.

Though background slowing, amplitude attenuation, and loss of reactivity are associated with increasing severity of encephalopathy, these features may not always occur in perfect sequence, nor do they precisely correlate with the bedside clinical examination. However, they collectively offer a useful overall assessment of the depth of encephalopathy, which may be trended over time using either follow-up EEGs or continuous monitoring. Reversal of these trends may indicate improvement.

Severe encephalopathies (such as traumatic brain injury or cerebral anoxia) are typically associated with slow, low-voltage, and unreactive electrographic patterns. However, an estimate of severity should not be confused with prognostication, as this is dependent on the etiology. A severe encephalopathy due to a reversible cause such as a medication-induced coma may have a similar electrographic appearance to anoxic brain injury (e.g., both may show burst suppression) but portend very different outcomes [5].

Identifying Repetitive Patterns and Understanding Their Implications

Generalized and lateralized repetitive abnormalities are commonly observed in encephalopathic patients; they're described in Chapter 15. Identification of these repetitive patterns has important implications regarding etiology, potential for epileptic seizures (epileptogenicity), neuronal injury, and prognosis. These points are discussed below.

Etiology: Though poorly specific, electrographic patterns are suggestive of the underlying etiological process. Generalized rhythmic delta activity (GRDA) and generalized periodic discharges with triphasic morphology (triphasic waves) are commonly observed in toxic-metabolic encephalopathies. Lateralized periodic discharges (LPDs) typically suggest an acute destructive process (such as herpes encephalitis), and generalized periodic discharges (GPDs) may be associated with nonconvulsive status epilepticus (NCSE).

Epileptogenicity: Common repetitive patterns that are strongly associated with epileptic seizures include lateralized rhythmic delta activity (LRDA), generalized periodic discharges (GPDs), bilateral periodic discharges (BIPDs), and lateralized periodic discharges (LPDs). Occipital intermittent rhythmic delta activity (OIRDA) may be associated with idiopathic generalized epilepsies, as shown in Figure 23.3.

Prognosis: Periodic patterns are electrographic markers of neuronal injury; consequently, they are associated with poor outcomes. However, it is not clearly understood if these patterns are merely the manifestation of neuronal injury or themselves have some causal role. Both GPDs and LPDs have been traditionally associated with increased mortality. Though recent studies do not show a direct association with increased mortality, GPDs are associated with NCSE, which itself is independently associated with increased mortality. Rarely, cyclical alternating patterns (CAP) may be seen in coma; these typically consist of alternating sequences of high-amplitude slowing with low-amplitude faster activity. They may represent state changes and are associated

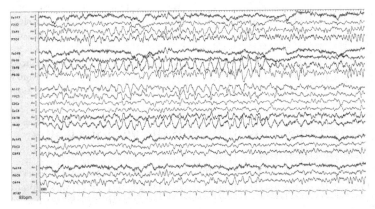

Figure 23.3 Eight-year-old boy with childhood absence epilepsy, runs of occipital intermittent rhythmic delta activity (OIRDA).

with favorable outcomes. However, it should be emphasized that etiology and not the electrographic pattern alone is the key determinant of clinical outcome [6,7].

Diagnosing Nonconvulsive Status Epilepticus

Rhythmic and periodic lie on an ictal–interictal continuum; at the ictal end they represent ongoing epileptic activity that is potentially contributing to the encephalopathic state without overt clinical signs – this is called nonconvulsive status epilepticus (NCSE). There are no universally accepted criteria for the diagnosis of NCSE. In practice, a diagnosis requires a combined assessment of clinical signs (altered mentation, aphasia, subtle motor, and behavioral signs) and EEG findings (continuous or recurrent electrographic ictal activity) that last 5 min or longer and may improve with a trial of antiepileptic medications. A diagnostic response to antiepileptics (such as lorazepam) must involve both clinical and electrographic improvement (resolution of ictal activity and crucially, return of normal background). These responses may be delayed or equivocal and not necessarily rapid, as described in Chapter 15. Timely identification of NCSE is important as it has been independently associated with increased mortality, and a diagnostic delay may contribute to worse clinical outcomes. NCSE is described in Chapter 24. Figure 23.4 shows NCSE.

Additionally, the reader must be familiar with a handful of "classical" electrographic presentations of encephalopathy with specific diagnostic

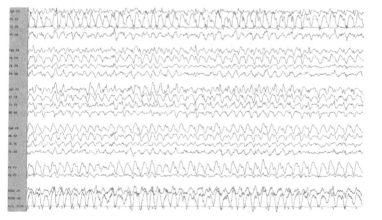

Figure 23.4 Twenty-seven-year-old woman with anti-NMDAR encephalitis, continuous generalized rhythmic discharges consistent with NCSE.

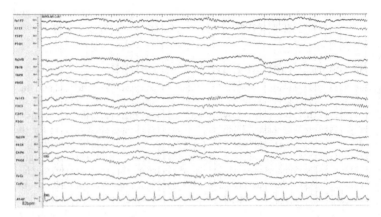

Figure 23.5 Thirty-six-year-old man with narcotic overdose, spindle coma pattern.

implications. These include spindle coma, alpha-theta coma, CJD, SSPE, and extreme delta brush.

Spindle Coma

The EEG is characterized by a diffuse theta and/or delta background with frequent 11- to 14-Hz symmetric spindles. On stimulation, K complexes may be seen along with other sleep architecture, such as vertex waves, however, clinically, the patient remains unconscious without arousals or fluctuations. Spindle coma is commonly associated with traumatic brain injury, drug overdoses, cerebral anoxia, and viral encephalitis. Anatomically, the pattern suggests involvement below the level of the thalamus, which is where spindles are thought to originate (such as Ponto mesencephalic junction). Prognosis is thought to be favorable depending on the presence of reactivity and absence of structural damage. If coma deepens, spindle frequencies may slow. Figure 23.5 shows a spindle coma pattern in the setting of a narcotic overdose [8].

Alpha/Alpha-Theta Coma

The EEG is characterized by mixed alpha and theta frequencies. There are a few distinct subtypes based on etiology:

1. Alpha coma associated with cerebral anoxia is characterized by diffuse or frontally predominant, monomorphic, unreactive alpha (continuous featureless alpha) with a grim prognosis (Chapter 25).

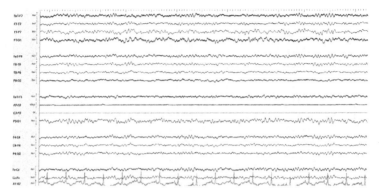

Figure 23.6 Forty-seven-year-old man comatose after pontine tumor removal, diffuse alpha activity (C3 electrode disabled).

2. Toxic metabolic encephalopathies (such as a drug overdose) are associated with mixed alpha and beta frequencies that show some reactivity and typically have a favorable prognosis.
3. Posterior-predominant alpha may suggest a pontine lesion. Alpha coma of pontine origin should be differentiated from a locked-in syndrome where the EEG resembles normal wakefulness with reactivity to sensory stimulation and photic driving. Continuous recording in those with locked-in syndromes will also reveal evidence of state change including sleep architecture (rapid and non–rapid eye movement sleep). These may be fragmented or diminished in appearance due to disruption of the reticular networks. Prognosis is typically poor, with high mortality. Figure 23.6 shows alpha coma pattern in pontine injury [9].

Beta Coma

The EEG is characterized by diffuse 12- to 16-Hz beta activity with a frontal predominance. Reactivity to sensory stimulation is usually preserved in lighter forms. Sedative-hypnotic overdoses are the most common cause, usually with favorable prognosis. Figure 23.7 shows diffuse beta activity in the setting of benzodiazepine overdose [10].

CJD and SSPE

These are two infectious pathologies with distinct electrographic patterns.

The EEG in Creutzfeldt–Jakob disease (CJD) is characterized by frequent (every 1 s) generalized periodic discharges with a di- or triphasic morphology.

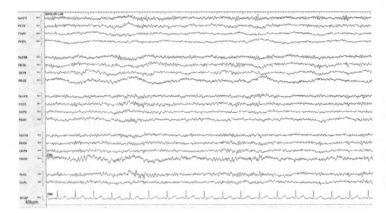

Figure 23.7 Twenty-eight-year-old woman with benzodiazepine overdose, diffuse excessive beta activity.

They may initially have a focal or lateralized predominance. The background is usually diffusely slow when the complexes first occur. Chapter 15, Figure 15.5 shows GPDs in CJD [11].

The EEG in subacute sclerosing panencephalitis (SSPE) is characterized by less frequent (every 4–14 s), high-amplitude, generalized periodic discharges (burst-like complexes) maximal in the frontocentral channels. Initially the background may be normal. The periodic complexes may be associated with myoclonic jerking (eyes or limbs), as shown in Figure 23.8 [12].

Extreme Delta Brush

Extreme delta brush is characterized by rhythmic (RDA) or periodic delta slowing with overriding bursts of rhythmic 20–30 Hz beta frequencies (plus fast features) that resemble beta-delta complexes in neonates. There is little reactivity or variability with sleep. This pattern, though nonspecific, has been described in many patients with anti-NMDA receptor encephalitis. Figure 23.9 shows extreme delta brush [13,14].

Chapter Summary

1. Global dysfunction (encephalopathy) results from impaired functioning of both cerebral hemispheres and/or brainstem.

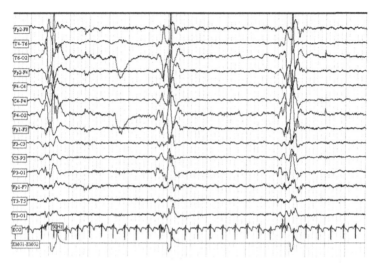

Figure 23.8 Five-year-old boy with SSPE, generalized periodic discharges associated with myoclonic jerks.

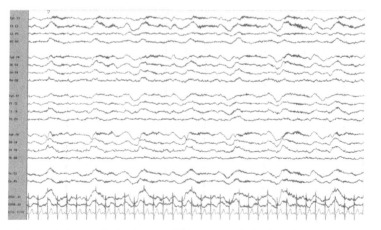

Figure 23.9 Same patient as in Figure 23.4, extreme delta brush pattern.

2. The EEG is an exquisitely sensitive tool to detect encephalopathy, but not specific to the underlying etiology.

3. The basic approach to an encephalopathic EEG consists of diagnosing encephalopathy, estimating its severity, and identifying repetitive patterns and NCSE, if present.

4. The three cardinal electrographic features of encephalopathy include background slowing, amplitude attenuation/suppression, and loss of reactivity.

5. Severe encephalopathies are typically characterized by a low-amplitude, slow and unreactive record, while a reversal of these trends may indicate improvement. Estimation of severity differs from prognostication.

6. Repetitive patterns (rhythmic and periodic) are common in encephalopathic patients and have important implications regarding etiology, epileptogenicity, and prognosis.

7. NCSE results from electrographic ictal activity that contributes to the encephalopathic state. It should be diagnosed based on clinical signs, EEG findings, and a response to antiepileptic medications. NCSE is independently associated with increased mortality.

8. Spindle coma is characterized by slow background with frequent symmetric spindles and typically has a favorable prognosis in those with reactivity and without evidence of structural damage.

9. Alpha coma consists of unreactive alpha frequencies; they have a posterior predominance in brainstem lesions and an anterior or diffuse distribution with cerebral anoxia. Posterior predominant alpha coma should be differentiated from a locked-in syndrome.

10. Beta coma typically occurs from drug overdose and usually has a favorable prognosis.

11. CJD and SSPE are infectious encephalopathies with distinct electrographic presentations that typically consist of GPDs.

12. Extreme delta brush pattern may suggest anti-NMDA receptor encephalitis.

References

1. Plum F, Posner JB. The diagnosis of stupor and coma. Oxford University Press, New York; 1982.

2. Kaplan PW. The EEG in metabolic encephalopathy and coma. Journal of *Clinical Neurophysiology*. 2004 Sep 1;**21**(5):307–18.

3. Hawkes CH, Bryan-Smyth L. The electroencephalogram in the "locked in" syndrome. *Neurology*. 1974 Nov 1;**24**(11):1015.

4. Sutter R, Stevens RD, Kaplan PW. Clinical and imaging correlates of EEG patterns in hospitalized patients with encephalopathy. Journal of *Neurology*. 2013 Apr 1;**260**(4):1087–98.

5. Young GB. The EEG in coma. *Journal of Clinical Neurophysiology*. 2000 Sep 1;**17**(5):473–85.

6. Kassab MY, Farooq MU, Diaz-Arrastia R, Van Ness PC. The clinical significance of EEG cyclic alternating pattern during coma. *Journal of Clinical Neurophysiology*. 2007 Dec 1;**24**(6):425–28.

7. Chong DJ, Hirsch LJ. Which EEG patterns warrant treatment in the critically ill? Reviewing the evidence for treatment of periodic epileptiform discharges and related patterns. *Journal of Clinical Neurophysiology*. 2005 Apr 1;**22**(2):79–91.

8. Kaplan PW, Genoud D, Ho TW, Jallon P. Clinical correlates and prognosis in early spindle coma. Clinical *Neurophysiology*. 2000 Apr 1;**111**(4):584–90.

9. Kaplan PW, Genoud D, Ho TW, Jallon P. Etiology, neurologic correlations, and prognosis in alpha coma. Clinical *Neurophysiology*. 1999 Feb 1;**110**(2):205–13.

10. Carroll WM, Mastiglia FL. Alpha and beta coma in drug intoxication. British *Medical Journal*. 1977 Dec 10;**2**(6101):1518.

11. Wieser HG, Schindler K, Zumsteg D. EEG in Creutzfeldt–Jakob disease. Clinical *Neurophysiology*. 2006 May 1;**117**(5):935–51.

12. Gökçil Z, Odabaşi Z, Aksu A, Vural O, Yardim M. Acute fulminant SSPE: clinical and EEG features. Clinical *Electroencephalography*. 1998 Jan;**29**(1):43–48.

13. Schmitt SE, Pargeon K, Frechette ES, et al. Extreme delta brush: a unique EEG pattern in adults with anti-NMDA receptor encephalitis. *Neurology*. 2012 Sep 11;**79** (11):1094–100.

14. Wang J, Wang K, Wu D, et al. Extreme delta brush guides to the diagnosis of anti-NMDAR encephalitis. *Journal of the Neurological Sciences*. 2015 Jun 15;**353** (1–2):81–83.

Status Epilepticus

Status epilepticus (SE) is a neurological emergency, it is practically defined as 5 min or longer of continuous clinical and/or electrographic seizure activity or recurrent seizure activity without recovery between seizures. The EEG plays a crucial role in the diagnosis, classification, and monitoring treatment of SE [1].

Conceptually, the International League Against Epilepsy (ILAE) suggests that SE results from the failure of mechanisms responsible for seizure termination or initiation of mechanisms which lead to abnormally prolonged seizures (after time point t1) with long-term consequences (after time point t2) that include neuronal injury, death, and alteration of neuronal networks. Hippocampal abnormalities such as atrophy may be evident on neuroimaging [2].

Operationally, the first time point (t1) indicates when emergency treatment of SE should be initiated as it is unlikely to spontaneously terminate beyond this time point and the second time point (t2) indicates when long-term consequences should be expected. The ILAE has published these time points for some types of SE. These general approximations are intended for operational use and based on experimental models; collaborative clinical evidence is emerging (see Table 24.1) [3].

Status epilepticus is described based on semiology (motor features), etiology (acute, remote, or progressive), electrographic features, and the age of occurrence.

Semiologically, it may be classified into two broad types:

1. *SE with prominent motor features:* This includes convulsive SE (CSE) and other less common forms such as focal motor status (epilepsia partialis continua and repetitive focal motor seizures/Jacksonian SE), tonic, clonic, and myoclonic SE.
2. *SE without prominent motor features (nonconvulsive SE):* This includes focal status with coma or impaired consciousness, absence status (may be typical, atypical, or de novo), aphasic status, and aura continua.

Etiologically, status epilepticus may be symptomatic of acute injury (such as a stroke or encephalitis), remote pathologies (such as poststroke or posttraumatic) or progressive conditions such as tumors or neurodegenerative

Table 24.1 Operational time points for status epilepticus

Type of SE	Time (t1) when a seizure becomes SE	Time (t2) when SE may cause long-term consequences
CSE (tonic clonic)	5 min	Greater than 30 min
NCSE (focal with impaired consciousness)	10 min	Greater than 60 min
NCSE (absence SE)	10–15 min	Unknown

disease. The electrographic features in SE are variable. Not all forms are associated with prominent electrographic correlates. Surface EEG findings are seen in only about 30% of those with pure motor seizures and 20% of those with nonmotor seizures without impaired awareness. Some forms of SE may be an integral part of age-dependent clinical syndromes [4].

Convulsive Status Epilepticus (CSE)

Convulsive status epilepticus may be generalized (GCSE) or more commonly focal onset with secondary generalization (focal to bilateral convulsive SE).

Clinically apparent CSE doesn't require an EEG for diagnosis. In fact, it may be significantly obscured by continuous (tonic phase) or regularly fragmented (clonic phase) myogenic/movement artifact as shown in Chapter 19, Figures 19.2 and 19.3. However, the EEG is crucial to differentiate mimics such as psychogenic status and other nonepileptic conditions with abnormal movements such as tremors, myoclonus, and dyskinesias. The EEG is diagnostic in situations where convulsive activity may not be apparent such as neuromuscular blockade. The EEG enables characterization and localization of ictal activity during CSE. After convulsions cease, it helps identify the cause of persistent altered mentation which may be secondary to sedatives, postictal encephalopathy, or ongoing ictal activity (NCSE) as shown in Figure 24.1. One study of 145 patients with CSE showed that about a third will evolve to NCSE [5]. Additionally, the EEG guides management including adjustments of sedation, instituting burst-suppression and monitoring for refractoriness or recurrence.

Initially, discrete electrographic seizures with interval slowing may occur, later these merges with waxing and waning ictal discharges or rhythmic ictal activity that may become continuous. Figure 24.2 shows focal status epilepticus while Figure 24.3 shows generalized status epilepticus.

As SE progresses, brief periods of suppression interrupt the continuous ictal activity as shown in Figure 24.4. Termination of ictal activity is typically

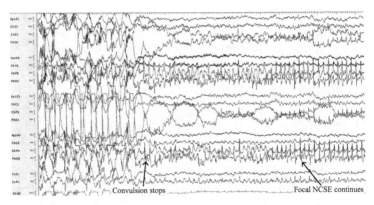

Figure 24.1 Twenty-seven-year-old woman with persistent postictal confusion, persistent right posterior temporal ictal activity consistent with NCSE.

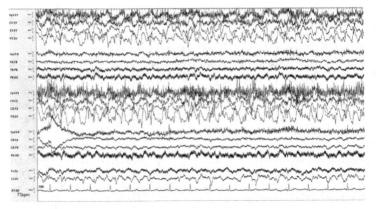

Figure 24.2 Forty-eight-year-old woman with CNS lymphoma, focal status epilepticus of left hemispheric onset.

characterized by generalized or lateralized periodic discharges, background suppression, and/or slowing with a gradual restoration of normal activities. Variations to these patterns are common and these stages may not follow in sequence. Cardiac rhythm disturbances such as ictal or postictal asystole may be noted on single EKG channel as previously discussed in Chapter 18 [6].

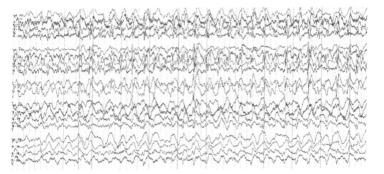

Figure 24.3 Same patient as in Figure 24.2, secondary generalized status epilepticus.

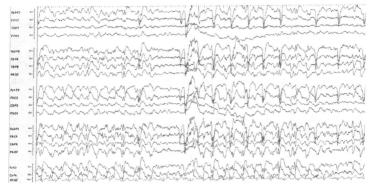

Figure 24.4 Fifty-six-year-old man with encephalitis, brief suppressions interrupt continuous ictal activity.

Nonconvulsive Status Epilepticus (NCSE)

Nonconvulsive SE is characterized by continuous or repetitive electrographic seizures without prominent motor features. Mentation may be affected to a variable degree ranging from subtle impairments in awareness or behavior to unresponsiveness and coma. This may occur following focal onset seizures that spread to impair awareness in ambulatory adults such as those with temporal or frontal lobe epilepsies, following CSE after convulsions have ceased or occur spontaneously in hospitalized and critically ill individuals with systemic and/or cerebral dysfunction

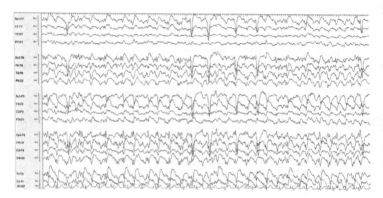

Figure 24.5 Same patient as in Figure 24.4, right hemispheric rhythmic polyspikes and wave discharges with wide fields consistent with focal onset NCSE.

who may not have a prior history of epilepsy. Since accompanying clinical manifestations may be subtle or absent, the EEG is crucial for diagnosis. Multiple studies have shown the incidence of NCSE to be at least 10–20% of those undergoing continuous EEG monitoring [7]. The diagnosis and clinical implications of electrographic seizures have been discussed in Chapter 16 (ictal patterns). Figure 24.5 shows NCSE.

Other Less Common Forms of Status Epilepticus

Epilepsia Partialis Continua (EPC)

Epilepsia partialis continua consists of focal onset motor SE (without impaired awareness) characterized by segmental myoclonus that may persist for prolonged periods. Common causes include strokes, malignancies, encephalitis, nonketotic hyperglycemia, or neuronal migration defects. The EEG is typically normal, electrographic changes occur in less than a third of patients and typically consist of focal discharges that correlate with contralateral motor movements as shown in Figure 24.6. This type of SE is often refractory to pharmacological treatments [8].

Absence Status

Absence SE may occur in three distinct forms:

1. *Typical absence SE:* This is seen in patients with idiopathic generalized epilepsies (IGE) such as CAE, JAE, or JME and is characterized by mild

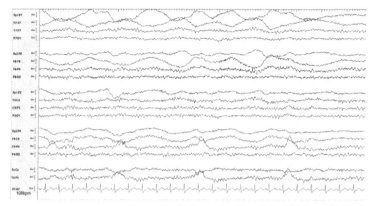

Figure 24.6 Fifty-nine-year-old woman with a right cortical stroke, focal right para-central (C4) blunted LPDs associated with repetitive left arm twitching.

impairments of awareness or confusional states, blinking, and occasional myoclonus that may persist for several hours. Sleep deprivation, alcohol, and benzodiazepine withdrawal are common triggers. A heralding convulsion may occur at the onset or terminate the event. EEG shows continuous generalized spike (polyspikes) and wave discharges up to 4 Hz in frequency with a frontal or central predominance. Spontaneous termination is not uncommon.

2. *Atypical absence SE:* This is relatively rare, typically occurring in infants and adolescents with underlying developmental deficits. Clinically it is characterized by confusion, subtle myoclonus, tonic, and atonic seizures. The EEG shows slow spike wave pattern and diagnosis typically requires careful comparison with prior studies.

3. *De novo absence SE:* This is characterized by confusion and is seen in older adults in the setting of abrupt withdrawals of benzodiazepines or other sleeping aids. Prior IGE may be present. EEG is like typical absence SE. Easily responds to treatment with benzodiazepines [9].

Tonic Status Epilepticus

Generalized Tonic SE is usually associated with Lennox–Gastaut syndrome (LGS). It is characterized by repetitive brief tonic contractions of the arms and extension of the legs. The EEG usually shows diffuse low-voltage fast activity, polyspikes, and slow waves as shown in Figure 24.7.

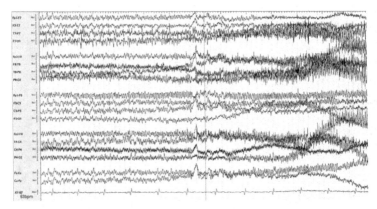

Figure 24.7 Thirty-one-year-old woman with LGS, continuous generalized low-amplitude fast activity associated with tonic status epilepticus.

Clonic Status Epilepticus

Generalized Clonic SE is usually seen in infants and children in association with febrile seizures or LGS. The EEG shows bilateral synchronous spikes, spiky bursts, and/or spike wave complexes.

Atonic Status Epilepticus

Atonic SE is usually seen in infants and children. It is clinically characterized by minor jerking, eye movements, and unresponsiveness. The EEG shows bilateral synchronous spike and slow-wave complexes. Prognosis is generally favorable.

Myoclonic Status Epilepticus

Myoclonus may be cortical (epileptic) or subcortical in origin (nonepileptic) In cortical myoclonus, myoclonic jerks are associated with epileptic discharges. Myoclonic status epilepticus refers to continuous epileptic myoclonus and potentially other seizure types. This is rarely seen in children with idiopathic generalized epilepsies (IGE) where the prognosis is usually favorable. This should be differentiated from myoclonic status epilepticus that occurs post cardiac arrest (sometimes referred to as status myoclonicus) which is typically associated with a poor prognosis. The EEG shows bilateral synchronous discharges associated with myoclonic artifact; these are best appreciated in the central channels that are relatively free of muscle artifact. Neuromuscular blockade may be selectively used to better appreciate epileptic discharges in those where the record is obscured with excessive myogenic artifact. Subcortical myoclonus such as metabolic myoclonus or that seen in posthypoxic syndrome (Lance Adam's syndrome) may not have reliable electrographic correlates [10]. Common electrographic patterns in cerebral anoxia are further described in Chapter 25.

Chapter Summary

1. SE is defined as 5 min or longer of continuous clinical and/or electrographic seizure activity or recurrent seizures without interval recovery.
2. A t1 refers to the time point beyond which there is failure of mechanisms responsible for seizure termination or initiation of mechanisms, which lead to abnormally prolonged seizures.
3. A t2 refers to the time point beyond which there are long-term consequences due to neuronal injury, death, and alteration of neuronal networks.
4. Semiologically, SE can be classified as with or without prominent motor features.
5. Convulsive SE may evolve into NCSE in a significant minority after convulsive activity ceases.
6. NCSE may be diagnosed on EEG in a significant minority of critically ill patients.
7. EPC may not be associated with ictal activity on surface EEG.
8. De novo absence SE may be seen in older individuals in the setting of abrupt benzodiazepine withdrawal. They may have a previous or family history of IGE.

References

1. Brophy G, Bell R, Alldredge A, et al. Neurocritical Care Society Status Epilepticus Guideline: guidelines for the evaluation and management of status epilepticus. *Neurocritical Care.* 2012;**17**:3–23.

2. Scott RC, King MD, Gadian DG, Neville BG, Connelly A. Hippocampal abnormalities after prolonged febrile convulsion: a longitudinal MRI study. *Brain.* 2003 Nov 1;**126**(11):2551–7.

3. Trinka E, Cock H, Hesdorffer D, et al. A definition and classification of status epilepticus – report of the ILAE Task Force on Classification of Status Epilepticus. *Epilepsia.* 2015 Oct;**56**(10):1515–23.

4. Verma A, Radtke R. EEG of partial seizures. *Journal of Clinical Neurophysiology.* 2006 Aug 1;**23**(4):333–9.

5. Yuan F, Yang F, Li W, et al. Nonconvulsive status epilepticus after convulsive status epilepticus: clinical features, outcomes, and prognostic factors. *Epilepsy Research.* 2018 May 1;**142**:53–7.

6. Pender RA, Losey TE. A rapid course through the five electrographic stages of status epilepticus. *Epilepsia*. 2012 Nov;**53**(11):e193–5.

7. Jette N, Claassen J, Emerson RG, Hirsch LJ. Frequency and predictors of nonconvulsive seizures during continuous electroencephalographic monitoring in critically ill children. *Archives of Neurology*. 2006 Dec 1;**63**(12):1750–5.

8. Thomas JE, Reagan TJ, Klass DW. Epilepsia partialis continua: a review of 32 cases. *Archives of Neurology*. 1977 May 1;**34**(5):266–75.

9. Thomas P, Lebrun C, Chatel M. De novo absence status epilepticus as a benzodiazepine withdrawal syndrome. *Epilepsia*. 1993 Mar;**34**(2):355–8.

10. Zhang YX, Liu JR, Jiang B, et al. Lance–Adams syndrome: a report of two cases. *Journal of Zhejiang University SCIENCE B*. 2007 Sep 1;**8**(10):715–20.

Chapter 25

Post Cardiac Arrest

A majority of patients with cardiac arrest remain unconscious despite successful restoration of spontaneous circulation. The EEG is useful to evaluate for nonconvulsive seizures and make prognostic estimations. It suppresses immediately following circulatory arrest but early electrographic improvements such as some restoration of physiologic rhythms (typically first 12 hours) is highly predictive of a favorable outcome whereas unfavorable patterns (called highly malignant patterns) are predictive of poor outcomes. However, the EEG alone isn't sufficient to reliably estimate outcomes in this critically ill population and it should be used in combination with other independent markers such as such as clinical examination (myoclonic SE, incomplete recovery of brainstem reflexes), bilateral absence of somatosensory evoked potentials (SSEPs) and/or neuroimaging as part of a multimodal approach [1,2].

Prior EEG based prognostication has been limited by the lack of a standardized classification system, interrater reporting variations, and confounding effects of therapeutic hyperthermia and sedation. Recently, there has been growing consensus on the definitions of electrographic patterns using standardized critical care EEG terminology that may reliably estimate prognosis in comatose patients after cardiac arrest [3].

These patterns are classified based on their prognostic significance as highly malignant, malignant, and benign. A recent multicenter study of routine EEGs of 103 comatose survivors recorded around 48 to 72 hours after cardiac arrest (upon rewarming) concluded that highly malignant patterns were 100% specific and about 50% sensitive for poor outcome (defined as best cerebral performance category score of 3–5 until 180 days). Individual malignant patterns had low specificity and sensitivity to estimate poor prognosis (around 48%) but if two malignant patterns were present then specificity for a poor outcome increased to 96%. Benign EEGs were predictive of favorable prognosis with a poor outcome present in only 1% of those patients. Additionally, therapeutic hypothermia and sedation did not significantly affect the pretest probabilities of electrographic patterns in this study. These results were corroborated by another study using continuous EEG showing background suppression and burst-suppression with identical bursts (highly malignant patterns) within 24 hours to be highly predictive of a poor outcome and recordings beyond 24 hours had no additional predictive value [3,4].

Approach to Electrographic Patterns Post Cardiac Arrest

1. Identify the electrographic pattern and understand their prognostic significance.
2. Identify nonconvulsive seizures.

Electrographic Patterns Post Cardiac Arrest

The EEG post cardiac arrest (cerebral anoxic injury) may be classified into one of the following three types:

1. *Highly Malignant EEG*: There is either suppressed background without discharges (Figure 25.1), suppressed background with continuous periodic discharges (Figure 25.2) or burst-suppression with or without discharges (especially with identical bursts) (Figure 25.3).
2. *Malignant EEG*: There may be malignant abnormalities of foreground, background, or reactivity. The presence of any two of these is highly specific for a poor prognosis.

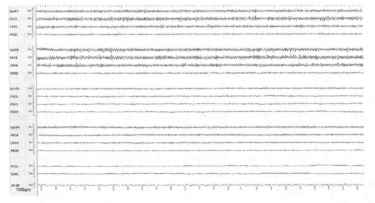

Figure 25.1 Seventy-eight-year-old man with cardiac arrest, suppressed background without discharges.

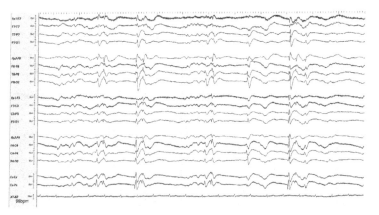

Figure 25.2 Sixty-two-year-old woman with cardiac arrest, suppressed background with continuous generalized periodic discharges.

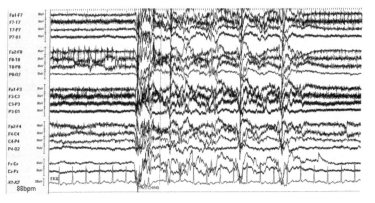

Figure 25.3 Seventy-eight-year-old man with cardiac arrest, burst-suppression (identical bursts) associated with myoclonic status epilepticus (time base of 20 s).

  a. foreground: periodic (Figure 25.4) or rhythmic discharges (Figure 25.5) and unequivocal electrographic seizures (ictal patterns)
  b. background: low voltage, discontinuity and/or reversals of anterior–posterior gradient (alpha-theta coma as shown in Figure 25.6)
  c. loss of background reactivity (or only stimulus-induced discharges)

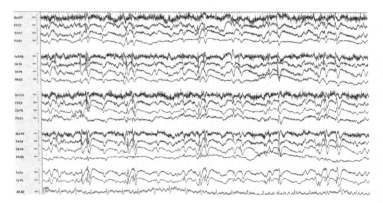

Figure 25.4 Sixty-seven-year-old woman with cardiac arrest, periodic discharges associated with myoclonic status epilepticus.

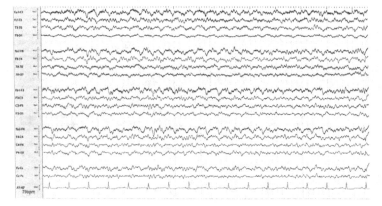

Figure 25.5 Fifty-seven-year-old man with cardiac arrest, generalized rhythmic delta with low amplitude sharps (GRDA plus S).

3. *Benign EEG*: No malignant features. This may predict a favorable outcome [3].

Seizures/Status Epilepticus Post Cardiac Arrest

Seizures and status epilepticus occur in about a third of patients who are comatose after cardiac arrest. They are typically nonconvulsive requiring

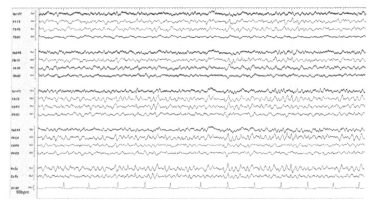

Figure 25.6 Fifty-four-year-old man with cardiac arrest, alpha-theta pattern with reversal of the anterior–posterior gradient.

continuous EEG monitoring for diagnosis. Seizures may be focal, generalized or multifocal in onset and tend to occur early during hospitalization or during rewarming [5]. Figure 25.7 shows NCSE post cardiac arrest. Status epilepticus post cardiac arrest is independently associated with increased mortality and continuous ictal activity may contribute to poor outcome [6].

Myoclonic SE is characterized by prolonged repetitive generalized or multifocal myoclonic jerking (often 30 min or more) that is time locked with bursts of burst-suppression (Figure 25.3) or associated with generalized periodic discharges (Figure 25.4). Early myoclonic SE (within 48 hours) from return of spontaneous circulation is highly predictive of poor outcome, though rare neurological recovery has been reported. The EEG is useful to identify reactivity and other signs of recovery in those with postarrest myoclonic SE after tapering off sedation [7].

Chapter Summary

1. EEG is useful to make prognostic estimations and evaluate for nonconvulsive seizures post cardiac arrest.
2. Unfavorable EEG patterns portend poor outcomes, whereas early improvements including restoration of physiological rhythms is associated with better outcomes.
3. The EEG has limitations; it should not be used in isolation to make prognostic estimations.

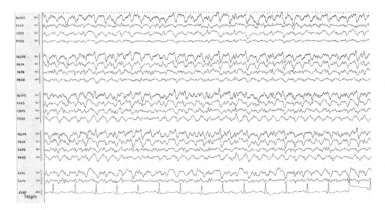

Figure 25.7 Same patient as in Figure 25.5, evolving generalized rhythmic sharp discharges consistent with NCSE.

4. Highly malignant EEG patterns are specifically associated with poor outcomes.
5. Individual malignant patterns have low sensitivity and specificity for poor outcomes.
6. Benign patterns (absence of malignant features) suggest favorable outcomes.
7. Seizures and status epilepticus are common post cardiac arrest and may contribute to poor outcomes.
8. Myoclonic status epilepticus is characterized by prolonged cortical myoclonus. Early myoclonic status epilepticus post cardiac arrest is typically associated with poor prognosis.

References

1. Crepeau AZ, Rabinstein AA, Fugate JE, et al. Continuous EEG in therapeutic hypothermia after cardiac arrest: prognostic and clinical value. *Neurology*. 2013 Jan 22;**80**(4):339–44.

2. Jehi LE. The role of EEG after cardiac arrest and hypothermia: EEG after cardiac arrest. *Epilepsy Currents*. 2013 Jul;**13**(4):160–1.

3. Westhall E, Rossetti AO, van Rootselaar AF, et al. Standardized EEG interpretation accurately predicts prognosis after cardiac arrest. *Neurology*. 2016 Apr 19;**86**(16):1482–90.

4. Hofmeijer J, Beernink TM, Bosch FH, et al. Early EEG contributes to multimodal outcome prediction of postanoxic coma. *Neurology*. 2015 Jul 14;**85**(2):137–43.

5. Rittenberger JC, Popescu A, Brenner RP, Guyette FX, Callaway CW. Frequency and timing of nonconvulsive status epilepticus in comatose post-cardiac arrest subjects treated with hypothermia. *Neurocritical Care*. 2012 Feb 1;**16**(1):114–22.

6. Rossetti AO, Logroscino G, Liaudet L, et al. Status epilepticus: an independent outcome predictor after cerebral anoxia. *Neurology*. 2007 Jul 17;**69**(3):255–60.

7. Sandroni C, Cariou A, Cavallaro F, et al. Prognostication in comatose survivors of cardiac arrest: an advisory statement from the European Resuscitation Council and the European Society of Intensive Care Medicine. *Intensive Care Medicine*. 2014 Dec 1;**40**(12):1816–31.

Brain Death

The American Academy of Neurology (AAN) recommends EEG as one of the ancillary methods used to confirm cerebral death in combination with a standardized clinical evaluation [1]. The EEG when recorded using the minimal technical standards as outlined by the American Clinical Neurophysiology Society's (ACNS) guidelines determines electrocerebral inactivity (ECI). Studies have shown that ECI corroborated a clinical determination of brain death in 96.5% of adults but similar findings have not been reproduced in children [2,3,4].

Electrocerebral inactivity (previously called electrocerebral silence) is defined as the absence of any nonartifactual (cerebral) activity over 2 uV (peak to peak) on a scalp EEG recorded using electrode pairs at least 10 cm apart and other technical criteria outlined by the ACNS.

ACNS Guidelines on minimal technical standards for EEG recording in suspected cases of cerebral death include the following recommendations [2]:

1. There should be a complete complement of scalp electrodes (including midline channels Fz, Cz, Pz which are relatively free of artifact and therefore useful to detect low-voltage cerebral activity).
2. Interelectrode impedances should be between 100 and 10,000 ohms to avoid distortion and amplification of extraneous signals.
3. The integrity of the entire recording system should be tested manually by touching each electrode with a pencil point or cotton swab to elicit artifact and verify the integrity of connections.
4. Electrode pairs should be at least 10 cm apart. Typically, the international 10–20 system has average adult interelectrode distances of 6 to 6.5 cm but increasing the interelectrode distance may show cerebral potentials otherwise not seen with usual sensitivities. The 10–10 system may also be used in addition to regularly used montages such as a central reference (Cz).
5. Use a sensitivity of 2 uV/mm for at least 30 min with adequate and appropriate calibration. Thirty minutes is recommended as intermittent suppressions may mimic ECI.

6. High-frequency (low pass) filter should not be set below 30 Hz and low-frequency filter (high pass) should not be above 1 Hz to avoid attenuation of low-voltage fast activity or slow frequencies. Avoid using a 60 Hz notch filter.

7. Additional monitoring techniques such as EKG, EMG, and hand channels help identify artifactual activity. Continuous video recording aids interpretation.

8. The absence of reactivity to intense somatosensory, auditory, and visual stimuli should be confirmed. Electroretinograms can persist in response to photic stimulation.

9. Recordings should only be performed by a qualified technologist.

10. If inconclusive, the EEG should be repeated in about 6–24 hours.

11. Physiological variables such as temperature, blood pressure, oxygen saturation, and medications (especially sedatives and narcotics) should be considered when interpreting ECI. A toxicology screen may also be obtained.

Chapter Summary

1. The EEG is recommended as an ancillary test to confirm brain death in combination with a standardized neurological examination.

2. The EEG must be recorded using specific technical parameters outlined by the American Clinical Neurophysiology Society (ACNS) to determine electrocerebral inactivity (ECI) which highly correlates with brain death.

3. Electrocerebral inactivity is defined as the absence of any nonartifactual (cerebral) activity over 2 uV (peak to peak) on a scalp EEG recorded using electrode pairs at least 10 cm apart and other technical criteria outlined by the ACNS.

References

1. Russell JA, Epstein LG, Greer DM, et al. Brain death, the determination of brain death, and member guidance for brain death accommodation requests: AAN position statement. *Neurology.* 2019 Jan 29;**92**(5):228–32.

2. Stecker MM, Sabau D, Sullivan LR, et al. American Clinical Neurophysiology Society guideline 6: minimum technical standards for EEG recording in suspected cerebral death. *The Neurodiagnostic Journal.* 2016 Oct 1;**56**(4):276–84.

3. Fernández-Torre JL, Hernández-Hernández MA, Muñoz-Esteban C. Non-confirmatory electroencephalography in patients meeting clinical criteria for brain death: scenario and impact on organ donation. *Clinical Neurophysiology.* 2013 Dec 1;**124**(12):2362–7.

4. Nakagawa TA, Ashwal S, Mathur M, Mysore M, Society of Critical Care Medicine. Guidelines for the determination of brain death in infants and children: an update of the 1987 Task Force recommendations. *Pediatrics.* 2011 Sep;**128**(3).

Appendix   How to Write a Report

It has been mentioned that a good report is one where the narrative is complete enough for the reader to picture the essentials of the original record. As with most neurological findings, it is best to describe what you see in simple terms rather than use convoluted terminologies and equivocations. The report will usually fall into the hands of a treating physicians who may not be a neurologist. Therefore, it becomes important to avoid EEG related jargon and if this is unavoidable, clearly explain the implications.

It is recommended that the report consists of three main parts:

1. introduction
2. description
3. interpretation

Introduction

This part should include the patient's name, demographics, and identifiers. It should briefly describe the reason for testing and prior preparations such as sleep deprivation, and it should list any relevant medications that may affect the EEG. This should be followed by a brief technical summary describing the system of electrode placement (e.g., standard 10–20 electrodes), any additional modifications, monitoring of other physiological parameters, and the commercial system in use. The total recording time may also be mentioned here.

Description

This is the main body text of the report. It should consist of objective descriptions of the predominant background and overlying foreground patterns, irrespective of whether they are normal or abnormal. Each physiological state during the recording should be described separately. Start with the description of the record during wakefulness followed by drowsiness and sleep. If a certain state was not achieved, then that should be mentioned. This should be followed by a description of the results of activation procedures such as hyperventilation and photic stimulation. If an event (such as a seizure) occurs during the recording, note the time of occurrence (or push button) and approximate duration. A concise description of the event should include the clinical semiology (either witnessed at bedside or on video), accompanying electrographic changes and heart rhythm on single EKG channel. The presence of significant artifact or EKG abnormalities should also be included. Avoid passing judgments about clinical significance in this part of the report.

Interpretation

This should consist of the reader's *impression*, that is, a subjective statement if the recording is normal or abnormal with relevant reasoning. If abnormalities occur, readers should further comment if they are epileptic or ictal. The record should also be compared to any prior studies, if these are available for review. Separately, a *clinical correlation* should also be attempted to explain how the reader's impression fits into the overall clinical picture. This should be carefully worded so as not to confuse the requesting clinician who may not be a neurologist. Further recommendations as may be relevant, such as longer duration of monitoring or repeating the study after sleep deprivation, can be included here [1].

Sample Normal Report

Routine EEG Report

Name:
Medical Record Number:
Date of Birth:

Reason: This is a 25-year-old man with no significant past medical history presents with episodes of tremulousness.

Relevant medications: none

TECHNICAL SUMMARY: This is a routine EEG performed with anterior temporal as well as standard 10–20 electrodes. Data are recorded using a Nihon Kohden ® digital EEG machine.

DETAILS: The waking background shows good organization, consisting of predominantly 30–40 μV, 9–10 Hz posterior background activity with good reactivity. There is moderate beta activity bilaterally.

Intermittent drowsiness is further characterized by attenuation of the background, slow roving eye movements, and bilateral slowing in the theta and delta range with shifting predominance. Stage N2 sleep is characterized by, further slowing, vertex sharp waves, sleep spindles, K complexes, and posterior occipital sharp transients of sleep (POSTS). Hyperventilation results in mild bilateral buildup. Photic stimulation results in mild bilateral driving. Single lead EKG shows an apparent sinus regular sinus rhythm.

IMPRESSION: This 30-minute routine EEG with video, performed in the waking, drowsy, and sleeping states is within normal limits. There are no definite epileptiform abnormalities or electrographic seizures during this record. There were no prior EEGs to compare.

CLINICAL CORRELATION: A normal EEG does not exclude the diagnosis of epilepsy.

Sample Abnormal Report
Routine EEG Report

Name:
Medical Record Number:
Date of Birth:

Reason: This is a 67-year-old man with past medical history of hypertension, depression, and peripheral neuropathy who is being evaluated for spells of impaired awareness.

Relevant medications: lisinopril, venlafaxine, cyanocobalamin tablets, and levetiracetam.

Indications: Assess epilepsy risk, interval EEG, now on antiepileptics.

Method: This recording was performed on XLTEK/Natus® equipment. Voltage filters were adjustable, applied as needed after recording. Standard 10–20 EEG electrode placement was used with additional anterior temporal electrodes as needed. The entire EEG dataset was reviewed by eye, with digital spike and seizure detection tools also employed.

DETAILS:

Artifact: Electrode artifact was mild. Myogenic artifact was mild. Artifact did not significantly degrade data quality.

Mental status: Awake and alert.

The waking background was well organized with appropriate posterior dominance and good reactivity to eye closure. The background was symmetric with an amplitude of 20–100 uV and predominant frequency of 9–10 Hz. Moderate beta activity was present bilaterally.

There were frequent brief bursts (1–5 s) of rhythmic, 50–200 uV, 2–2.5 Hz slowing seen over the left temporal region (F7, T1, T3). Additionally, there were occasional independent bursts (1–3 s) of higher amplitude (75–300 uV), polymorphic, bitemporal, 1–3 Hz delta slowing.

Drowsiness demonstrated frontocentral slowing, attenuation of the posterior-dominant rhythm and accentuation of above mentioned slowing. Brief sleep demonstrated further slowing, vertex waves, central spindles, and K complexes. Later stages of sleep were not seen.

Hyperventilation was not performed. Photic stimulation demonstrated moderate driving.

Single EKG channel demonstrated a normal sinus rhythm of 60–80 beats per minute.

Impression: This 30-minute routine EEG with video is abnormal due to the following features:

1. Frequent bursts of left temporal rhythmic slowing consistent with temporal intermittent rhythmic delta activity (TIRDA) which has

a high association with mesial temporal lobe epilepsy (epileptogenic abnormality).

2. Occasional independent bitemporal slowing accentuated during drowsiness and light sleep.

These findings are unchanged in comparison to a prior EEG.

Clinical correlation: This study is consistent with left temporal cortical irritability (seizure tendency) and mild, left greater than right, bitemporal dysfunction. The study captured no events. There were no electrographic seizures during this study.

A Few Sample Interpretations for Reference

"This routine EEG, performed in wakefulness, drowsiness, and slight sleep shows no definite abnormalities. Bilateral irregularities are noted mostly during drowsiness, perhaps right greater than left which do not clearly exceed normal limits for drowsiness. Infrequent wickets are noted and considered a benign pattern of uncertain significance."

"This routine EEG, performed in the waking, drowsy, and sleep states is abnormal because of bilateral left greater than right hemispheric slowing and rare left sharp waves. This study is consistent with moderate left hemispheric dysfunction and cortical irritability (seizure tendency) in the setting of a mild encephalopathy. A breach rhythm is noted over the left frontotemporal region consistent with his known craniotomy."

"This portable EEG performed on a patient in the obtunded state is abnormal due to continuous bilateral hemispheric slowing and abundant generalized periodic discharges (GPDs) with a triphasic morphology (also called triphasic waves). This study is consistent with moderate to severe encephalopathy to which medications and/or metabolic dysfunction may contribute."

"This portable EEG performed on a patient in the confused state reveals

1. Frequent electroclinical seizures with P3 onset, and at times associated with right arm clonic jerking, right gaze deviation, and altered awareness. They occur at a frequency of 8–10 per hour without improvement in the patient's mental status between seizures, consist with nonconvulsive status epilepticus (NCSE). Seizures stop after intubation at 17:30.

2. Frequent lateralized periodic discharges (LPDs) in the left frontal-central region and isolated discharges over the right parietal region in the initial part of the record.

3. Continuous high-voltage delta slowing over the left side throughout the initial part of record.

4. Predominantly poorly organized, discontinuous, and slow background with burst-suppression of the record after intubation and resolution of NCSE."

These findings are suggestive of seizures and focal cortical irritability over the left parietal region and left more than right bi-hemispheric cerebral dysfunction. Seizures stop and are replaced by a burst-suppression pattern following intubation and initiation of sedation. The higher voltage on the left side is consistent with a breach artifact due to known skull defect. A prior EEG on -- showed left greater than right hemispheric slowing, with no seizures."

"This routine EEG performed in the waking and drowsy and states is abnormal because of frequent bursts of generalized epileptiform discharges as described. These findings are indicative of interictal expression of generalized epilepsy syndrome."

"This routine EEG performed in the waking and excessive drowsy states shows no significant abnormalities. Excessive drowsiness without evidence of sleep may suggest sleep deprivation. An event tremulous involuntary limb and body movements as noted by the technologist during the study is not associated with a definite epileptiform correlate."

Summary

1. Always treat the patient and not the EEG. Epilepsy is a clinical diagnosis where the EEG is but a single data point.
2. Ideal reports are those that clearly state if the recording is normal or abnormal with appropriate reasoning.
3. Confusing or entirely unexpected findings should arouse suspicion.

Reference

Kaplan PW, SR. Benbadis How to write an EEG report: dos and don'ts. *Neurology*. 2013 Jan 1;80(1 Supp 1): S4 3–6.

Index

Printed in the United States
by Baker & Taylor Publisher Services